The Eye in General Practice

C. R. S. Jackson
MA DM (Oxon) DOMS FRCS (Edin)
Formerly Consultant Ophthalmic Surgeon, Royal Infirmary, Edinburgh and Clinical Tutor in Ophthalmology, University of Oxford

R. D. Finlay
MA BM BCh (Oxon) FRCS FRCS (Edin) DO FCOphth
Consultant Ophthalmic Surgeon, Royal United Hospital, Bath and formerly Postgraduate Clinical Tutor, Bath Health District

NINTH EDITION

CHURCHILL LIVINGSTONE
EDINBURGH LONDON MELBOURNE NEW YORK AND TOKYO 1991

CHURCHILL LIVINGSTONE
Medical Division of Longman Group UK Limited

Distributed in the United States of America by Churchill Livingstone Inc., 1560 Broadway, New York, N.Y. 10036, and by associated companies, branches and representatives throughout the world.

First edition 1957
Second edition 1960
Third edition 1964
Fourth edition 1967
Fifth edition 1969
Sixth edition 1972
Seventh edition 1975
Eighth edition 1985
Ninth edition 1991
Reprinted 1992

ISBN 0-443-04381-7

British Library Cataloguing in Publication Data
Jackson, C. R. S. (Charles Robert Sweeting)
The eye in general practice.–9th ed.
1. Man. Eyes. Diseases
I. Title II. Finlay, R. D. (Robin Dundas)
617.7

Library of Congress Cataloging in Publication Data
Jackson, C. R. S. (Charles Robert Sweeting)
The eye in general practice/C. R. S. Jackson, R. D. Finlay. — 9th ed.
p. cm.
Includes index.
ISBN 0–443–04381–7
1. Ocular manifestations of general diseases. 2. Eye — diseases and defects. 3. Family medicine. I. Finlay, R. D. II. Title.
[DNLM: 1. Eye Diseases. 2. Eye Manifestations. WW 100 J12e]
RE65.J34 1991
617.7 — dc20
DNLM/DLC
for Library of Congress
90–2381
CIP

The publisher's policy is to use **paper manufactured from sustainable forests**

Produced by Longman Group (FE) Ltd
Printed in Hong Kong

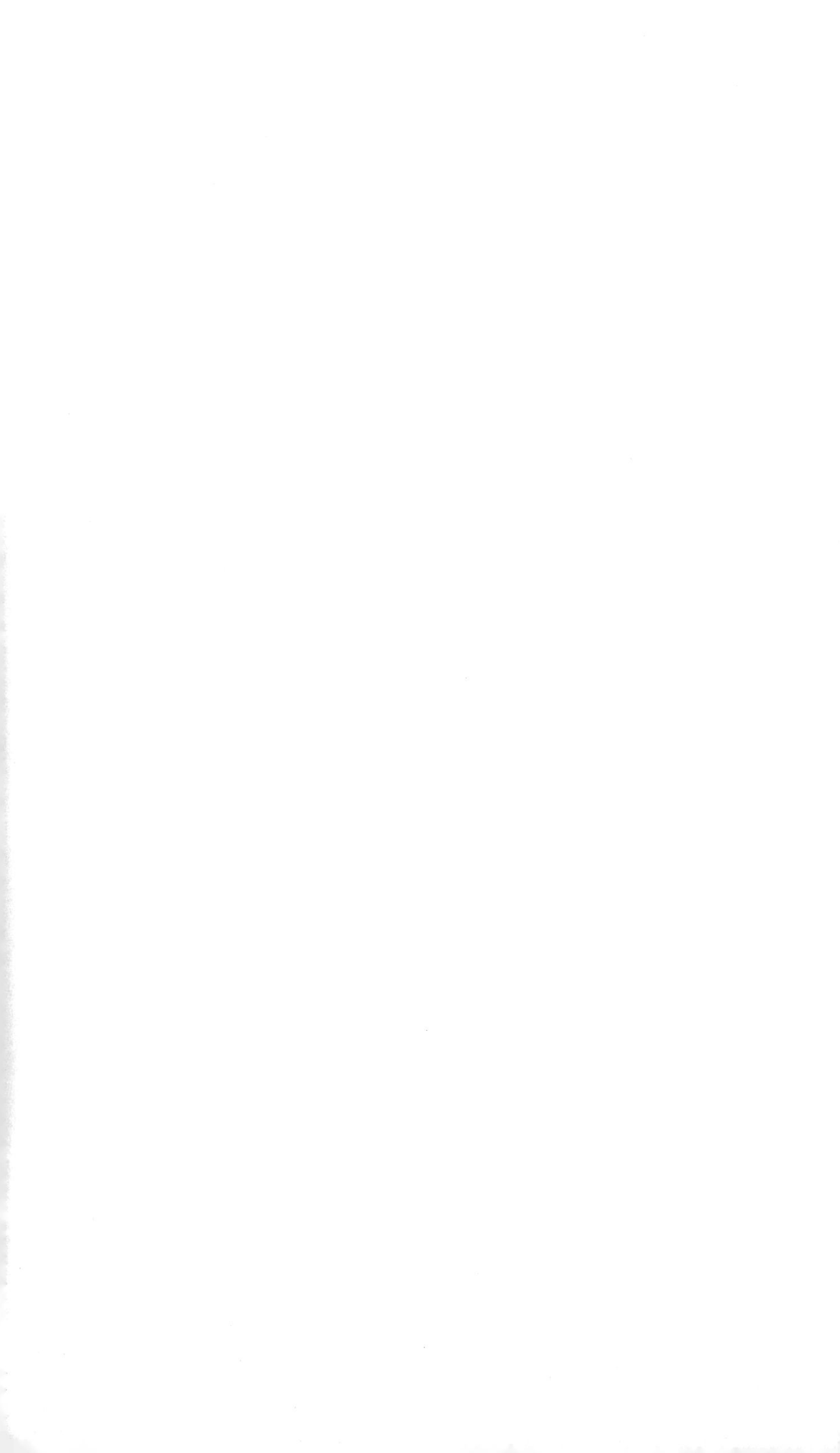

Preface

The average general practitioner sees about three patients a week with eye problems and yet most doctors' own perceptions of their knowledge and skills in ophthalmology remain low. The time devoted to the subject in the undergraduate curriculum and that of the post-graduate vocational trainee in general practice is severely restricted.

Perhaps the most effective way for a trainee to gain greater proficiency is to attend hospital eye clinics on a regular basis for a few weeks; but a textbook which sets out the commoner problems clearly and concisely is required. The authors hope that this new edition will serve the needs both of the undergraduate and of the general practice vocational trainee, and also those of the established general practitioner.

The format of the completely rewritten eighth edition has been retained. There is an introductory chapter on the methods of history taking and examination, and a second, setting out, on a problem-orientated basis, the differential diagnosis of the commoner symptoms presented by a patient to the general practitioner. Changes in the text reflect developments in ophthalmology in the past five years.

Emphasis continues to be placed on those conditions which a general practitioner will treat himself, and on those for which a patient may expect an informed assessment and appropriate referral. This applies particularly to the problem of diabetic retinopathy.

The text has, in places, been expanded in response to helpful comments from some teachers in an attempt more fully to supply the needs of medical students.

It is the authors' hope that this book will earn a place on each general practitioner's bookshelf and, perhaps, on those of ophthalmic nurses, orthoptists, ophthalmic opticians and others concerned with the care of the visually handicapped.

Acknowledgements

The authors are indebted to many colleagues for their advice and, in particular, to Messrs J. D. Griffiths and D. E. P. Jones, and to Drs J. Heber, S. Lenton, P. G. Mann, J. P. D. Reckless, R. D. Thomas and Diana White, all of Bath. Also to Messrs J. McGill of Southampton and J. Marsh of London. They are also deeply grateful to colleagues who have kindly provided illustrations: Dr T. Barrie of Glasgow, Mr D. L. Boase of Portsmouth, Professor S. Darougar of London, Miss Elizabeth Eagling of Birmingham, Professor D. L. Easty and Mr C. Dean Hart of Bristol, Mr J. Kanski of Windsor, Mr R. S. Mahto of Bath, Mr S. P. B. Percival of Scarborough, Mr G. J. Romanes of Dorchester, Dr N. L. Stokoe of Edinburgh, and Mr J. D. Strong of Swindon; also to the Consultant Radiologists at Bath.

Mr R. Wm. Mackie, of The Society for Welfare and Teaching of the Blind (Edinburgh and S.E Scotland), helped us to find sources of information, as did Miss Alison Stephenson, Librarian at The Royal College of Surgeons of Edinburgh.

Messrs Clement Clarke and Messrs Keeler kindly allowed us the use of illustrations.

For the Medical Photographers at the Royal United Hospital, Bath, Ms Alex Morefield and Miss Samantha Ellis, nothing appears to have been too much trouble.

C. R. S. J.
R. D. F.

Contents

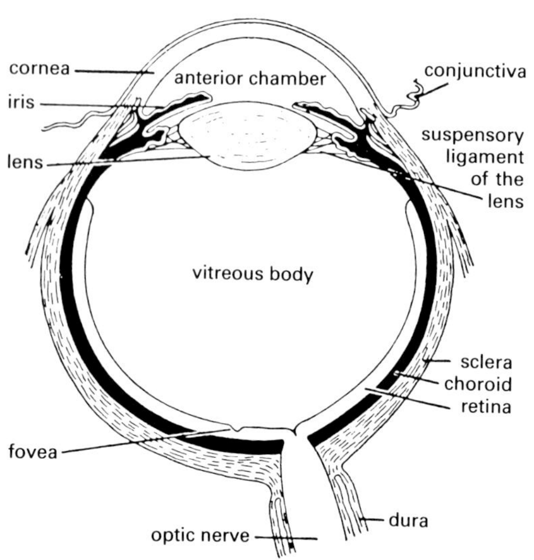
cornea
anterior chamber
conjunctiva
iris
suspensory
ligament
of the
lens
lens
vitreous body
sclera
choroid
retina
fovea
dura
optic nerve

1. History and examination

Between 1 and 2% of patients attending general practitioners' surgeries do so on account of symptoms related to their eyes, so some attempt must be made to help in sorting out the various problems.

There may be pain, redness, watering, alteration in appearance, impaired or double vision. It must not be forgotten that some with disease of the eye or visual pathway have no complaint.

There may be a history of previous similar episodes, of systemic illness, of eye disease in the family; and the way in which symptoms first present may give us clues. In particular, bilaterality or otherwise is important. A complaint of sudden visual loss may represent a sudden appreciation of a long-standing defect — as, for example, on happening to close or cover the 'good' eye.

Possible injury must not be overlooked — especially industrial injury through hammering, drilling, and so on. The nature and distribution of the pain may be important. The 'scratchy' pain of a superficial foreign body is quite distinct from the pain of deeper eye disease, which is often referred to brow or cheek, through the trigeminal nerve.

An adequate initial examination of the eye can be made with simple apparatus.

The following are the minimum requirements:

1. Pen torch. Held between finger and thumb, the disengaged fingers resting on the patient's face and helping to keep the eye open (Fig. 1.1).
2. Magnifier (×8). For maximum field of view it must be held close to the examiner's eye.
3. Fluorescein-impregnated paper strips (Fluorets®) moistened with the tears in the lower part of the conjunctiva (Fig. 1.2). (NB Never use fluorescein in bottles — danger of contamination, espe-

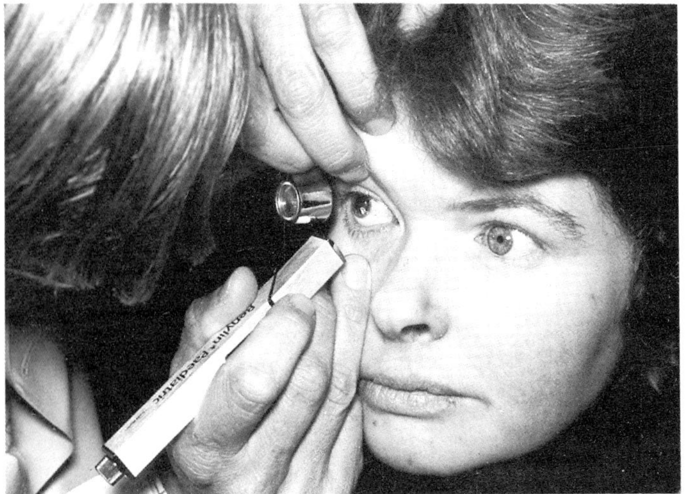

Fig. 1.1 Examination with torch and loupe

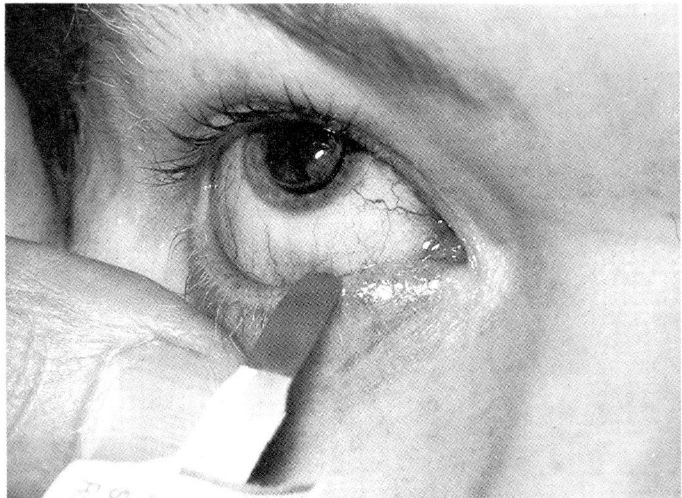

Fig. 1.2 Staining with fluorescein

cially by *Pseudomonas*). An alternative to fluorescein is rose bengal. A corneal epithelial defect will pick up the stain; green (fluorescein) or red (rose bengal).

4. Quick-acting, short-lasting mydriatic, to dilate the pupil if need be. Useful drugs are homatropine 2%, cyclopentolate 0.5 or 1.0% (Mydrilate®), and tropicamide (Mydriacyl®) 0.5 or 1.0%. These are available in disposable, single-dose containers (Minims-SNP). Atropine should be avoided, its effects being unnecessarily prolonged.

After the examination, a drop of pilocarpine 2% counteracts the effect of the mydriatic. (Mydriasis = dilation of the pupil. Miosis = pupillary constriction.)

5. Ophthalmoscope. Several general practitioner models are available — more useful if the battery is fresh and the bulb not blackened with age. A darkened room makes examination easier.

The use of the ophthalmoscope with a +20 lens in place is valuable as an alternative means of examining the anterior segment of the eye if pen torch and loupe are not available.

Methods

The first thing to do — and often overlooked — is to test the vision in each eye separately, with glasses if worn, for both distance and reading. (Some patients put on their reading glasses when invited to 'read' the distance test type!) Make sure that the eye not under test is adequately covered. Children, especially, are liable to 'peek'.

The Snellen (Fig. 1.3) line labelled '6' can be read by the normal eye at 6 m — hence 6/6. Diminishing ability is represented by 6/9, 6/12, and so on. A test card for near vision is useful, but a newspaper or telephone book will serve. For young children, and those who cannot read, some kind of illiterate test is needed. Letter matching tests such as the Sheridan Gardiner (Fig. 1.4) or Stycar are most frequently used. The child identifies a letter at 3 or 6 m and matches it with one of a number of letters on a card held in his hand. Most children of 3 years or older can manage this test (see p. 5).

If the patient has no glasses — or has left them at home — the 'pin-hole' test may be of help. An eye in which defective vision is due to refractive changes or other 'anterior segment' problems will almost invariably have much improved vision when peering through a small hole punched in a piece of dark card. Plenty of light — and a steady hand — will be required, especially in the elderly, but the satisfaction of demonstrating that the central retina is intact is significant.

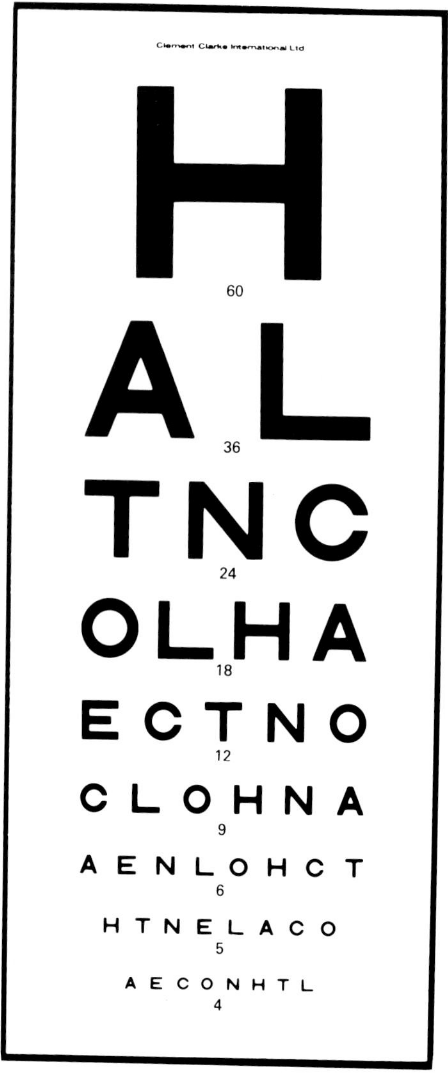

Fig. 1.3 Snellen test type (6 and 3 metre versions available)

Visual fields

The test of visual acuity takes account only of central vision. For completeness, a test of peripheral vision may be made by sitting in front of the patient and comparing the extent of his peripheral

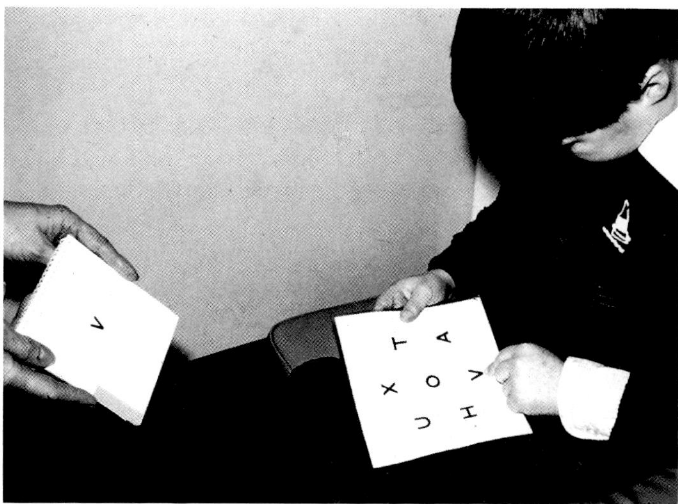

Fig. 1.4 Sheridan Gardiner test

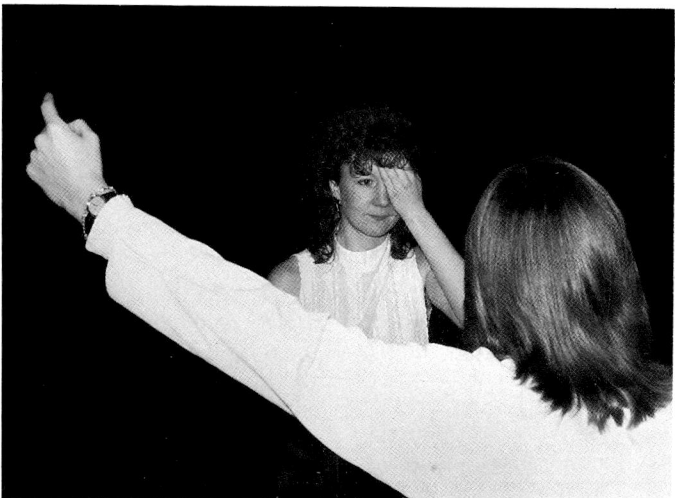

Fig. 1.5 Confrontation test for visual field

visual field with one's own, examining the eyes separately (Fig. 1.5).

At least, the ability to detect the movement of a hand in each of the four quadrants should be checked. This visual field test may

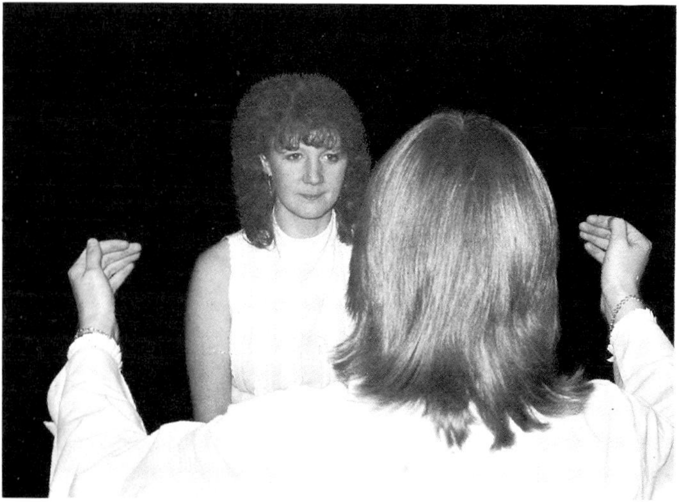

Fig. 1.6 Test for hemianopia

reveal hemianopia from damage to the visual pathways, or field loss from glaucoma, both of which may exist in the presence of normal visual acuity, the patient being unaware of the defect.

A homonymous defect is most readily demonstrated by the examiner facing the patient and using both hands (Fig. 1.6). Failure to see either hand indicates hemianopia; the defect is confirmed by moving the unseen hand across the midline, whereupon the patient is able to see both. This simple test should be repeated in the upper and lower quadrants.

It may be helpful to ask the patient to count the examiner's fingers in different quadrants of the visual field where there is doubt about a defect.

Eyelids

Symmetry on the two sides is to be expected. Drooping or over-elevation of the upper lid may point to ptosis or lid retraction, perhaps from palsy of the oculomotor nerve or from dysthyroid eye disease.

The skin around the eye is examined, and the normal position of the eyelashes. Inflammation of the lid margin may be noted, or swellings in the lid substance.

The surface of the eye

The patient must keep both eyes open. If this is difficult, a drop of short-acting local anaesthetic is invaluable — amethocaine 1% or oxybuprocaine (Benoxinate) 0.4%.

Redness most marked on the lining of the lids and around the periphery of the eye — conjunctivitis — is differentiated from that which is duskier in colour and seen mostly around the margin of the cornea — ciliary congestion — suggesting disease of the cornea, iris, or deeper parts of the eye.

In the examination of the outer eye, the bright shiny surface of the cornea will be noted. Defects will be identified after the use of stain — see above.

Pupils

The normal pupils are round, central and of equal size: they react equally to light and accommodation. Examination requires four simple steps:

1. *Inspection*. Look for any irregularity of size, shape or position of either pupil.

2. *Light reaction*. With the fellow eye covered, shine the brightest light available — it may be a pen torch, ophthalmoscope or desk light — directly into each eye in turn. A brisk, sustained contraction should be seen, the pupil dilating when the light is removed. The pupil of the eye not exposed to the light should constrict to the same extent — this is the consensual reaction.

3. *The swinging light test*. Illuminate first one eye and then the other. Each should show an equal and similarly sustained pupil reaction. Dilatation of either pupil when illuminated indicates impaired conduction along the optic nerve on that side — a relative afferent pupillary defect. This is a simple and sensitive test of optic nerve function.

4. *Near response*. The patient is instructed to look into the distance and then at an object held close to his face; both pupils constrict, dilating again when distant gaze is resumed. The near response is invariably present if the light reflex is normal. Only in the absence of a pupillary light reaction is a near response of relevance — 'light–near dissociation' (p. 154).

Abnormalities are discussed on page 153.

Colour vision

Colour vision testing is sometimes of importance to the general practitioner. Two circumstances in which assessment can be of value require different equipment:

1. *In optic nerve disorders* (Ch. 14) impaired colour recognition, especially of red, is an early finding. The colour may appear to be 'washed out' (desaturated), compared with its appearance when seen with the other eye. Red recognition is easily checked against that of the examiner by the confrontation test described for the visual field (Fig. 1.5), using a red target. A red-topped pin or a small red plastic bottle top is satisfactory.
2. *Congenital colour blindness* occurs in various forms in about 8% of males and 0.4% of females, with sex-linked recessive inheritance. Detection of this defect is useful in routine visual screening, and patients sometimes ask to be tested. Specially designed tests are used for occupational testing, as for airline and railway staff.

The *Ishihara* test is convenient for the general practitioner. It consists of a book of coloured plates, each bearing a number that the patient has to identify.

Ocular movements

A complaint of double vision should lead to the movement of an object in various directions, to find the direction in which double vision is present (see Fig. 12.5).

The inner eye

Only practice can bring competence with the ophthalmoscope. The closer to the eye the instrument is held, the wider the field of view. The use of a plus lens in the ophthalmoscope, and examination at 0.3 m, make for easier detection of lens opacities (Fig. 1.7).

It is important to examine both eyes, for asymmetry between the eyes is unusual and should make the alarm bells ring. Particularly with regard to the optic disc, differences between the two sides, of shape, size, colour, or of the vascular pattern, may be of crucial importance.

Be systematic when examining the fundi. One way is to look slightly to the nasal side, focus on a vessel and follow it until the

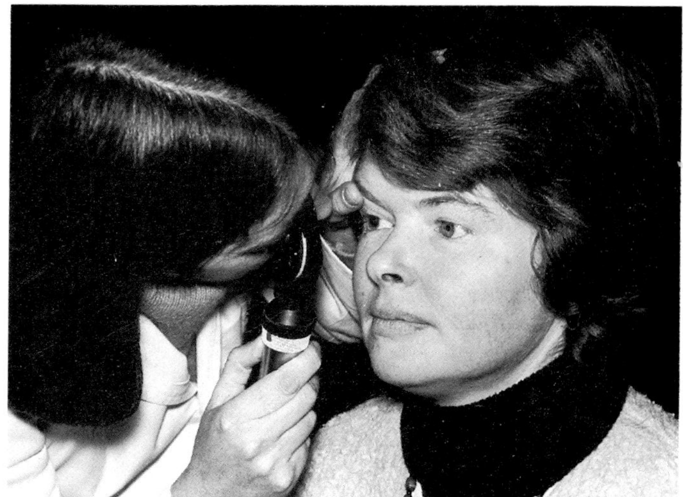

Fig. 1.7 Use of ophthalmoscope

optic disc is seen. The disc is then examined and each of the four main vascular arcades followed peripherally in turn. Finally the macula is examined; this may require a small aperture in the ophthalmoscope if the pupil has not been dilated.

2. Initial assessment

Symptoms have been discussed in Chapter 1. The remainder of the text is arranged on an anatomical basis and the purpose of this chapter is to draw the two parts together, while reminding the reader that serious disease of the eye or visual pathway may exist in the absence of symptoms.

Common presentations include:

1. Red eye
2. Pain
3. Visual loss — sudden or gradual
4. Distorted vision
5. Haloes
6. Flashing lights
7. Spots before the eye.

1. *The red eye.* Most cases of 'red' eye can be dealt with at the first visit. Cases of doubt should be referred for initial diagnosis and treatment by an ophthalmologist, urgently if vision is affected (Table 2.1).

2. *Pain in the eye.* This may arise in the eye or be referred from elsewhere. Cases of persistent pain in the eye should be referred for urgent examination by an ophthalmologist (Table 2.2).

3. *Sudden loss of vision.* Visual loss may be total or partial, affecting only a sector of the visual field; it may be transient, or may persist. Unequivocally diagnosed migraine is the only category in which urgent referral to an ophthalmologist is not mandatory. Patients over 60 who have sudden visual loss must have an immediate ESR or plasma viscosity check to detect asymptomatic giant cell arteritis. Missing this diagnosis may result in visual loss in the second eye and total blindness which could have been pre-

Table 2.1 The red eye

Condition	Symptoms	Signs	Management
Sub-conjunctival haemorrhage (p. 36)	No pain Normal vision	Haemorrhage visible Cornea clear	No treatment required
Conjunctivitis (p. 37)	Watery or purulent discharge Slight or no pain Normal vision	Conjunctiva inflamed	Antibiotic drops if bacterial infection suspected
Keratitis (p. 53)	Pain and photophobia Vision impaired if ulcer or opacity near visual axis	Loss of corneal clarity Epithelial defect stains with fluorescein	Antibiotic drops if bacterial infection clearly established — otherwise refer
Iritis (p. 65)	Pain Photophobia Vision may be impaired, or increase in floaters	Small or distorted pupil Ciliary congestion Engorged vessels radiating from limbus Tarsal conjunctiva normal	Refer for confirmation of initial diagnosis Treat recurrences with steroid drops and refer for follow-up
Acute glaucoma (p. 134)	Pain ±Vomiting Severe visual impairment May be bilateral	Pupil fixed and semidilated Corneal oedema preventing clear view of iris detail Shallow anterior chamber Raised intraocular pressure	Refer urgently
Episcleritis (p. 46)	Slight or no pain No discharge Normal vision	Localised or diffuse redness of bulbar conjunctiva and underlying episcleral tissues, which may be elevated.	Steroid drops, provided cornea is clear. Usually settles without treatment
Scleritis (p. 46)	Deep-seated pain	Localised or diffuse redness and swelling of sclera Frequently associated with systemic connective tissue disorder	Refer

Each of these conditions is considered in more detail and illustrated in the following chapters.

Table 2.2 Pain attributed to the eye

	Condition	Features
Major painful eye disorders	Cornea Keratitis (p. 53) Abrasion (p. 51) Foreign body (p. 52)	Ciliary congestion; fluorescein staining
	Iritis (p. 65)	Ciliary congestion; small, irregular pupil; vision may be impaired
	Scleritis (p. 46)	Usually associated systemic disorder
	Acute glaucoma (p. 134)	Corneal oedema; fixed, semi-dilated pupil; shallow anterior chamber; hard eye; may be vomiting
Eye disorders causing discomfort	Lids Entropion (p. 24) Trichiasis (p. 24)	Malpositioned or loose lashes
	Conjunctiva Conjunctivitis (p. 37) Dry eye (p. 31)	Palpebral and bulbar conjunctiva inflamed; discharge; Rose bengal punctate staining; Schirmer's test
	Episcleritis (p. 46)	Nodular or diffuse
	Optic neuritis (p. 147)	Vision impaired; colour recognition defective; afferent pupillary defect; discomfort on palpating globe and lateral gaze; may be disc swelling
Pain referred to the eye	Trigeminal nerve	
	Herpes zoster ophthalmicus (p. 56)	Rash
	Trigeminal neuralgia	Lancinating pain; trigger zone
	Sinusitis	Tender on pressure over sinus; X-ray
	Scalp (p. 146) Giant cell arteritis	Tenderness; raised ESR/plasma viscosity; may lead to sudden visual loss (ischaemic optic neuropathy)
	Neck Tension headache	Continuous, symmetrical pain; not associated with visual or gastrointestinal symptoms
	Intracranial	
	Migraine	Aura; distribution; duration; gastrointestinal symptoms
	Migrainous neuralgia	'Cluster' incidence; unilateral associated lacrimal and nasal discharge

continued overleaf.

Table 2.2 *(contd)*

Condition	Features
Raised intracranial pressure (p. 149)	Papilloedema; nausea/vomiting; headache worse in morning and on coughing/straining
Intracranial aneurysm	Associated cranial nerve lesion
Refractive error (p. 114)	Symptoms suggest eyestrain Refer for refraction in first instance
Ocular muscle imbalance (p. 128)	

vented. The principal causes of sudden loss of vision are given in Table 2.3.

4. *Gradual loss of vision.* The commonest causes are given in Table 2.4.

5. *Distorted central vision:*

   a. Retinal detachment beginning to involve macula (p. 98)
   b. Macular degeneration of any type (p. 88)
   c. Macular haemorrhage.

Pupillary light reaction is normal. Dilatation of the pupil is essential for satisfactory examination.

6. *Haloes round lights may be due to:*

   a. Raised intraocular pressure in angle-closure glaucoma (p. 135)
   b. Corneal disease
   c. Lens opacities.

Always refer for investigation to exclude angle-closure glaucoma.

7. *Flashing lights* before one or both eyes — the patient may not be sure — may be due to:

   a. Scintillating scotoma of migraine
   b. Retinal tear (p. 98)
   c. Retinal detachment (p. 98)
   d. Vitreous detachment.

Unless the history of migraine is certain, refer for detailed retinal examination.

Table 2.3 Sudden loss of vision

Site	Cause	Features
Vitreous	Massive vitreous haemorrhage (p. 87)	Loss of red reflex on fundus examination
Retina	Retinal arterial occlusion (p. 84)	Branch — partial loss of vision Central — total loss of vision and of direct pupillary reaction
	Central retinal vein occlusion (p. 86)	Extensive haemorrhage in fundus
	Amaurosis fugax (p. 85)	'Curtain' over vision, usually recovering in minutes. Embolism may be visible in retinal arteriole. Carotid bruit may be present
	Retinal detachment involving macula (p. 98)	Flashing lights, 'floaters', and visual field loss spreading centrally
Optic nerve	Ischaemic optic neuropathy (p. 147)	a. 'Anterior ischaemic' — usually partial visual loss and disc swelling b. Giant cell arteritis — disc swelling. ESR/viscosity raised
Visual pathway	Stroke (p. 151)	Homonymous hemianopia (the patient may think it unilateral). Total visual loss if previous hemianopia unrecognized or cortical blindness. Normal pupil reactions
	Migraine	Characteristic aura and recovery. Scintillating scotoma: flashing lights. Gastrointestinal symptoms. Recovery almost invariable
Acute glaucoma		Pain ± vomiting. Red eye. Corneal oedema. Semidilated pupil. Eye stony hard
Toxic reactions		Quinine or methyl alcohol poisoning

NB Apparently sudden loss of vision may be due to the discovery of a pre-existing defect or to hysteria. Referral is always justified.

Table 2.4 Gradual loss of vision

	Cause	Features
Lens	Cataract (p. 71)	Increased myopia or blurring
Retina	Macular degeneration (p. 88)	Straight lines appear distorted Peripheral field unaffected.
	Retinal vein occlusion (p. 86)	Typical retinal haemorrhages
	Retinal detachment (p. 97)	Flashing lights and 'floaters'. Visual field loss spreading centrally
Optic nerve	Chronic glaucoma (p. 136)	Usually so gradual as to pass unnoticed. Optic disc cupping, raised intraocular pressure and field loss
	Optic neuritis (p. 147)	Age group 20–45. Central field defect — peripheral field intact. Eye tender on palpation and on looking sideways. Impaired direct pupillary light reaction (p. 7). Spontaneous recovery usual in 2–4 weeks
	Toxic optic neuropathy	Heavy smoking and/or alcohol intake. Peripheral field intact
Visual pathway	Compressive lesions of visual pathway	Must be excluded if no other cause found. Temporal field defect usual. CT scan required

8. *Spots before the eyes:*

   a. Vitreous haemorrhage
   b. Uveitis with vitreous opacities (p. 66)
   c. Retinal tear with operculum lying in the vitreous (p. 98)
   d. Posterior vitreous detachment occurring suddenly
   e. 'Innocent' degenerative changes in the vitreous (p. 81)

This list contains enough vision-threatening conditions to justify referral if the general practitioner is not entirely satisfied that the condition is due to innocent vitreous opacities.

Flashing lights and spots before the eyes are a particularly dangerous combination — referral essential.

REFERRALS

Except in emergency, when contact is likely to be made by telephone, the majority of patients referred will have been examined initially by an optician. The sight-testing optician will send a letter or a completed proforma to the doctor. This report contains details of the optician's findings, and it should be sent complete to the ophthalmologist with the referral letter.

The optician's report will record the visual acuity, the spectacle correction and other findings. If this information is available to the ophthalmologist, repetition of some tests will be avoided and the point of the optician's referral will not be missed.

Also of importance are details of the patient's general state of health, with information about relevant past illnesses and family history. These are especially helpful with elderly patients who may not be good historians. A recent blood pressure reading and the result of a urine test for glucose will also be appreciated.

3. The eyelids

ANATOMY

The skin of the lid is thin and without subcutaneous fat. Inflammation or trauma leads to much swelling.

The margin of the upper lid normally crosses the upper third of the cornea, and the lower lid margin lies at the lower limbus (junction of cornea and sclera). Exposure of sclera below the cornea is one of the first signs of proptosis.

The tarsal or Meibomian glands lie in the substance of the lid and discharge at the lid margin.

In front, the lids have two or three rows of lashes, while the inner end of each lid carries the lacrimal punctum, the upper end of the lacrimal drainage apparatus, invisible unless the lid is everted.

The orbicularis muscle, supplied by the facial nerve, encircles the orbit and is responsible for blinking and for forced protective closure of the eye. The levator of the upper lid is supplied by the third cranial nerve.

WOUNDS OF THE LIDS

These injuries require special attention, because they may accompany an injury to the eyeball. Lid wounds are best treated in a specialist unit, as the distortion resulting from incorrect alignment may lead to unsightly notching of the lid margin, distortion of lashes or interference with lacrimal drainage.

Destructive injuries of the lids may expose the cornea, which must on no account be allowed to become dry. Pending repair, the cornea should be protected by the use of plenty of ointment and a pad.

INFLAMMATION OF THE LIDS

Blepharitis (inflammation of the lid margins) (Fig. 3.1)

This gives rise to chronically irritable eyes; the lid margins are reddened and conjunctivitis is present. Crusts are seen at the roots of the lashes. Seborrhoea capitis seems to be a common association. Treatment is tedious. Antibiotic ointment at night may help, with a short course of combined antibiotic–steroid for exacerbations if necessary. The crusts should be removed with a moistened cotton wool 'bud' before applying ointment.

Hordeolum (stye)

An abscess in one of the glands related to a lash follicle. Pointing, therefore, occurs in the line of the lashes, distinguishing this condition from the chalazion.

Treat by hot bathing and antibiotic ointment.

SWELLINGS OF THE LID

Benign

Chalazion (meibomian, tarsal, cyst) (Fig. 3.2)

A chronic swelling in the substance of the lid, painless unless abscess formation occurs. Characteristically centred some distance from the lid margin and thus distinguished from a stye.

Chalazia are often multiple and repeated, and are common in association with rosacea. Treatment consists of incision and curettage. This is an out-patient procedure which a general practitioner may wish to undertake.
The equipment required is:

Chalazion clamp
Chalazion curette
Fine scissors and forceps
Scalpel (No. 11 or 15 blade)
Anaesthetic drops (Amethocaine 1% or Oxybuprocaine 0.4%)
Local anaesthetic for injection
Antibiotic ointment
Eyepad.

Technique: Anaesthetize the conjunctiva with drops. Inject 1–2 ml of 1–2% lignocaine around the swelling — through the skin

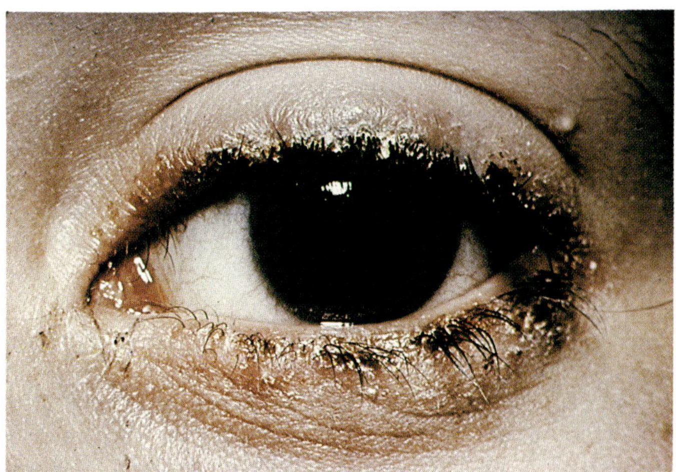

Fig. 3.1 Blepharitis

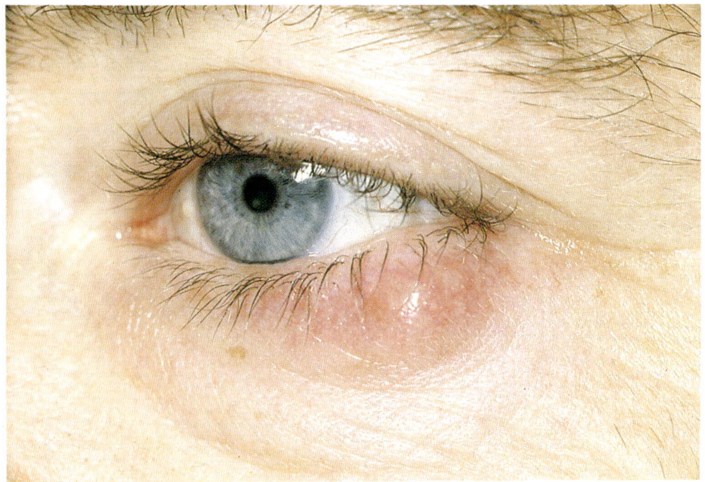

Fig. 3.2 Chalazion (tarsal cyst)

surface. Apply the clamp so that the cyst protrudes through the ring on the conjunctival side. Open the cyst through an incision at right angles to the lid margin, and curette out the (usually gelatinous) contents. It may be necessary to excise granulation tissue with scissors and forceps. Instil antibiotic ointment and apply a firm pad (over the closed eye). Local pressure should be maintained for 10 min or so. The pad can then usually be dispensed with. The eye should be bathed, and ointment instilled, twice daily for about 3 days.

Other cysts

Sebaceous cysts and molluscum contagiosum (Fig. 3.3) need surgical evacuation.

Xanthelasma (Fig. 3.4)

Common in the elderly and in diabetics, these flat creamy plaques may be removed on cosmetic grounds. They may signify hyperlipidaemia.

Malignant

Basal-cell carcinoma (rodent ulcer) (Fig. 3.5)

Characteristic rolled edges; typically seen in Europeans who have been exposed over many years to bright sunlight. The commonest malignancy in the eyelid; slow growing and only locally invasive.

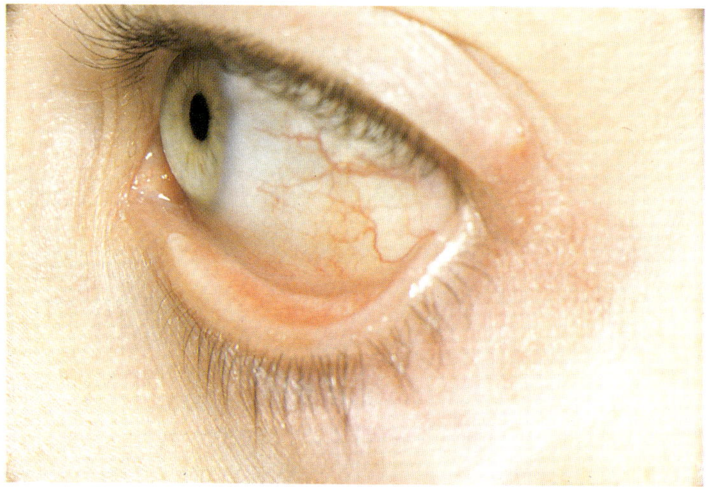

Fig. 3.3 Molluscum contagiosum — conjunctivitis associated with lesion on upper lid

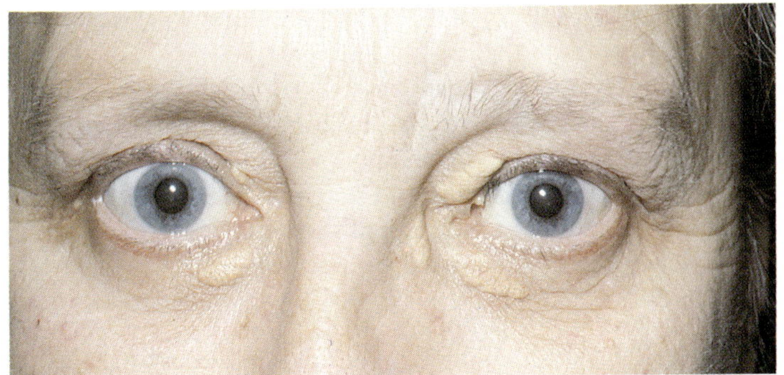

Fig. 3.4 Xanthelasma

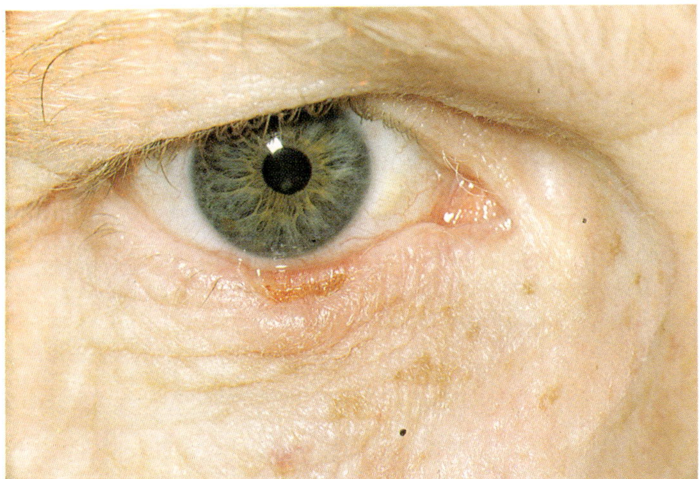

Fig. 3.5 Basal cell carcinoma (rodent ulcer)

If untreated, it leads to considerable loss of tissue. Treatment is by local excision with 2 mm of surrounding tissue, radiotherapy or cryotherapy, depending on the size and site of the lesion.

Squamous carcinoma (epithelioma)

Requires wide excision with diagnostic biopsy.

MALPOSITIONS OF THE LID

Trichiasis

Trichiasis is misdirection of the eyelashes and may result from wounds or inflammation. The abnormal lashes rub against the globe, with irritation, watering and potential damage to the cornea.

Treatment is difficult; simple epilation may suffice, or the offending lashes can be eliminated by electrolysis.

Entropion (Fig. 3.6)

A backward rolling of the lid edge, the lashes actually disappearing from view, occurs mostly in the elderly and is a result of spasm of the inner fibres of the orbicularis oculi (senile spastic entropion). It may occur spontaneously or follow irritation. If intermittent, entropion may be induced by asking the patient to close the eye forcibly. Temporary relief can be obtained by the use of a strip of plaster between the lid and the cheek, but recurrent or persistent entropion needs surgery. Refer.

Ectropion (Fig. 3.7)

The edge of the lower lid may fall away from the eye as a result of wounds or inflammation, but most commonly in facial palsy or senile loss of tone in the facial muscles.

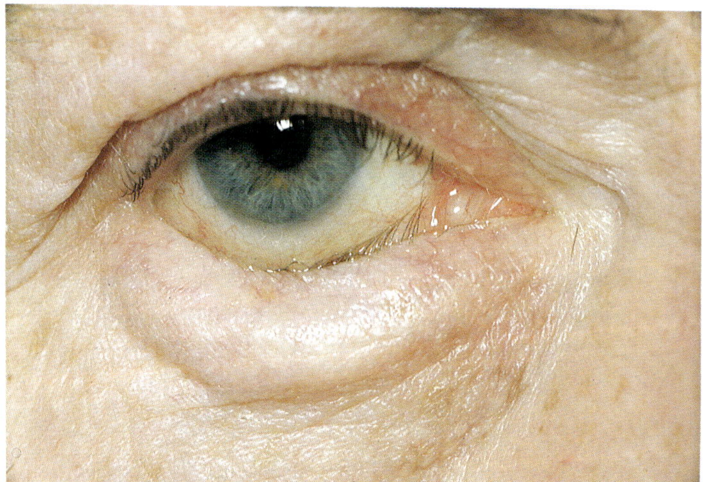

Fig. 3.6 Entropion

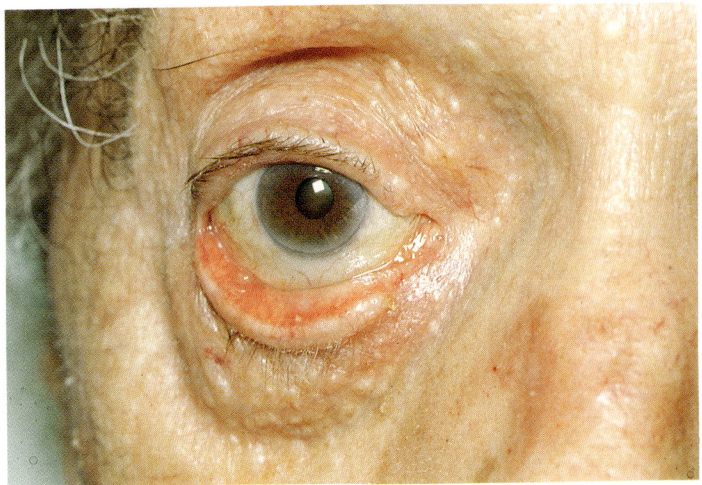

Fig. 3.7 Ectropion

The principal complaint will be of watering. Later there will be conjunctivitis and increased discharge.

Treatment is surgical, but the patient should be taught not to make the condition worse by wiping his eyes downwards. He should wipe his eye upwards and medially towards the nose.

Ptosis (Fig. 3.8)

Drooping of the upper lid occurs in palsy of the third cranial nerve and may result from a multitude of neurological conditions. It is a diagnostic sign of myasthenia gravis, and may be induced or made worse by asking the patient to gaze steadily at a finger held in front of his face and above the horizontal plane.

Of greater importance from the ophthalmic point of view is congenital ptosis, unilateral or bilateral, complete or partial. It is often associated with limited elevation of the affected eye, from weakness of the superior rectus muscle. It is impossible to mistake a child suffering from bilateral congenital ptosis, with the characteristic 'head back' attitude in his attempt to see through the reduced palpebral aperture. Treatment is surgical, and the timing of the operation depends on the child's age and whether or not there is a risk of the eye becoming amblyopic ('lazy') from disuse.

Congenital ptosis is sometimes associated with epicanthus (Fig.

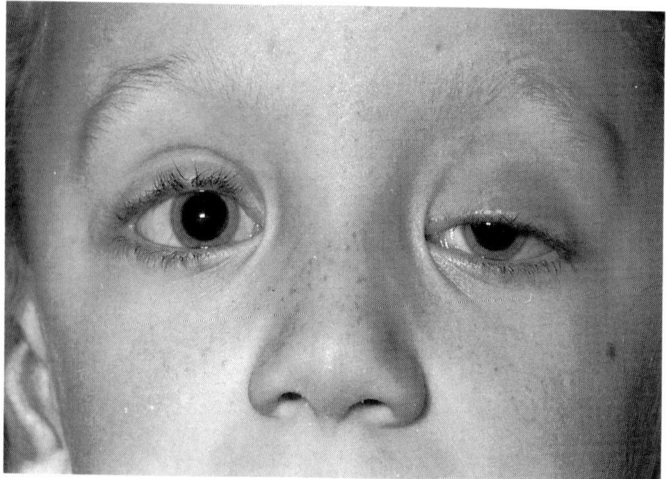

Fig. 3.8 Congenital ptosis

12.2, p. 125), a prominent fold of skin overlying the inner corner of the eye. This usually improves with age.

Senile ptosis is not uncommon, and a minor degree of ptosis constitutes part of Horner's syndrome (see p. 154).

DRUG SENSITIVITY REACTIONS

Allergic conjunctivitis with dermatitis involving the skin around the eyelids sometimes occurs. Drugs, notably neomycin and sulphacetamide, and some cosmetics, may cause a similar reaction. The intense irritation may be relieved by 1% hydrocortisone lotion.

FACIAL PALSY

Idiopathic facial palsy (Bell's palsy) may lead to exposure keratitis. In the early stage this is best prevented by applying ointment — usually containing an antibiotic such as chloramphenicol — liberally to the eye at night. If the eye becomes inflamed or corneal damage is demonstrated, the patient should be referred. Joining the lids by lateral tarsorrhaphy protects the cornea.

INVOLUNTARY MOVEMENT

Recognized as an everyday occurrence in response to injury or threat of injury, forcible closure of the eye is so common as to appear scarcely worthy of mention. When, however, blepharospasm occurs without warning and in the presence of a normal eye, it may become a matter of serious concern.

A degree of fibrillary twitching in one or more of the facial muscles is probably universal, and may amount to no more than a mild embarrassment, particularly when unilateral. Bilateral involuntary closure of the eyes, with temporary total blindness as a result, requires treatment.

Selective denervation of the orbicularis muscle is the treatment of choice, most readily achieved by injection of minute quantities of botulinum toxin into the muscle. The injection may be expected to give relief for up to 6 months, and can be repeated.

BLEPHAROPLASTY

This is a term used to describe a number of cosmetic surgical procedures to correct laxity of the eyelid skin. Complications may occur and the surgeon has an obligation to ensure that eye and adnexal disorders are evaluated before undertaking treatment.

4. The lacrimal system

ANATOMY AND PHYSIOLOGY (Fig. 4.1)

The lacrimal gland lies in the upper outer corner of the orbit and drains into the conjunctival sac. The tears are carried by movements of the lids to the inner corner of the eye. On each lid, at the inner end, is a minute lacrimal punctum, invisible until the lid is everted.

Two canaliculi carry the tears to the lacrimal sac, from which the nasolacrimal duct drains to the inferior meatus of the nose.

The conjunctiva is normally moistened by mucous and accessory lacrimal glands, the lacrimal gland providing extra lubrication when needed.

THE WATERY EYE

Abnormal watering (epiphora) is caused by overproduction of tears or interference with outflow.

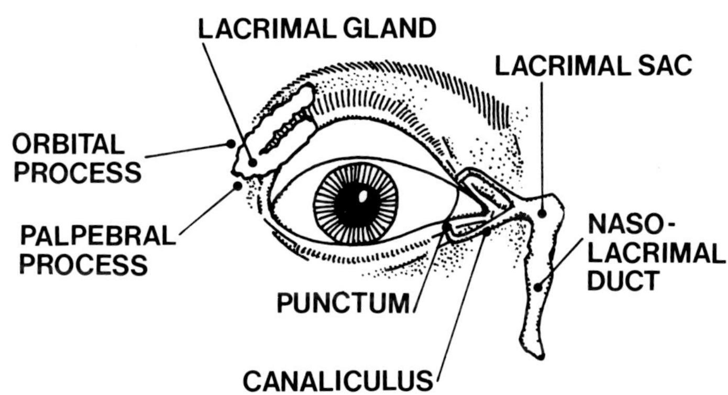

Fig. 4.1 Diagram of lacrimal apparatus

Epiphora from overproduction of tears

1. Irritation of conjunctiva or cornea, as by a conjunctival or corneal foreign body, or conjunctivitis.
2. Reflex epiphora from irritation of the fifth cranial nerve. Also, in some people, from exposure to bright light.

Epiphora from failure of outflow

1. Malposition of the punctum, which then fails to pick up the tears.
2. Occasionally, a loose lash gets washed into the punctum giving a characteristic patch of redness where it rubs against the conjunctiva. Removal of the lash produces a gratifyingly rapid cure.
3. Obstruction in the canaliculus: canalicular blockage is a rare cause of epiphora: it sometimes follows trauma.
4. Obstruction in the nasolacrimal duct:

   a. *In infancy*. The commonest cause of unilateral conjunctivitis in a baby. The nasolacrimal apparatus develops from a solid cord of ectodermal cells folded into the face along the groove between the frontonasal and maxillary processes. Subsequent canalization leads to the formation of the lacrimal sac and nasolacrimal duct. In some cases canalization is incomplete. There is no abnormality during the first weeks of life, and then the eye becomes watery and tends to be sticky. Finger pressure over the lacrimal sac may produce a reflux of mucoid material from the punctum. Conservative treatment is worthwhile for a few weeks. The child's mother is instructed to keep the sac empty by finger pressure several times a day, antibiotic drops being used at the same time. Many cases resolve spontaneously, but failure to do so is an indication for probing of the duct — an out-patient procedure under general anaesthetic.

   b. *In the adult*. Chronic obstruction of the nasolacrimal duct is often due to dacryocystitis, more common in women than in men, and mostly after the menopause. Chronic dacryocystitis leads to constant watering of the eye and may be associated with the development of a mucocele from which mucopus can be expressed by finger pressure over the sac. Not only is the obstructed duct liable to acute inflammation, it is also a reservoir from which infected material constantly enters the conjunctival sac. This means that any injury to the eye is liable to become infected, and any operation is similarly at risk. In most cases treatment is by the creation of a new channel to the nose. Dacryocystorhinostomy (DCR) consists of making an anastomosis between the lacrimal and nasal mucous membranes. The tears can then enter the nose, bypassing the obstructed nasolacrimal duct. Drops containing zinc sulphate 0.25% are available for the symptomatic relief of epiphora, used on a 'p.r.n.' basis.

THE DRY EYE

Inadequate tear production is an important cause of ocular discomfort and contributes to many cases of failure to tolerate contact lenses. Tear secretion naturally decreases with advancing age. The patient complains of vague irritation and attacks of redness of the eyes. The symptoms are variable, and tend to be worst in centrally heated buildings, and in cars with the heater blowing hot air.

Patients with collagen disorders, particularly rheumatoid arthritis, are prone to a more severe form of keratoconjunctivitis sicca, characterized by diminished tear and salivary secretion, with dryness of the cornea and formation of filaments on its surface (Sjögren's syndrome).

Tear production is assessed by Schirmer's test (Fig. 4.2). A strip of filter paper 5 mm wide is placed over the margin of the lower

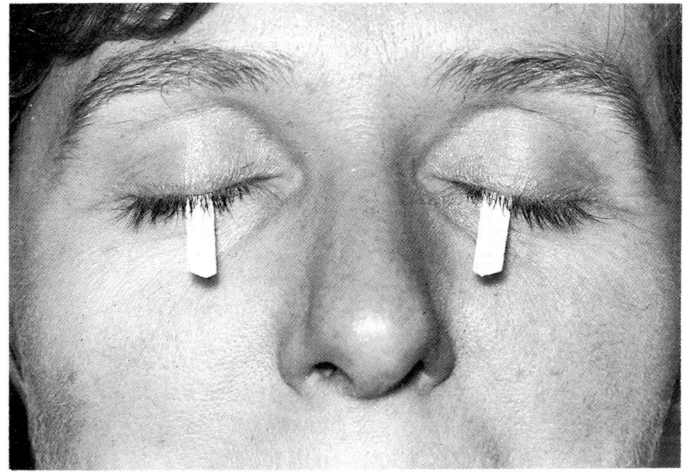

Fig. 4.2 Schirmer's test

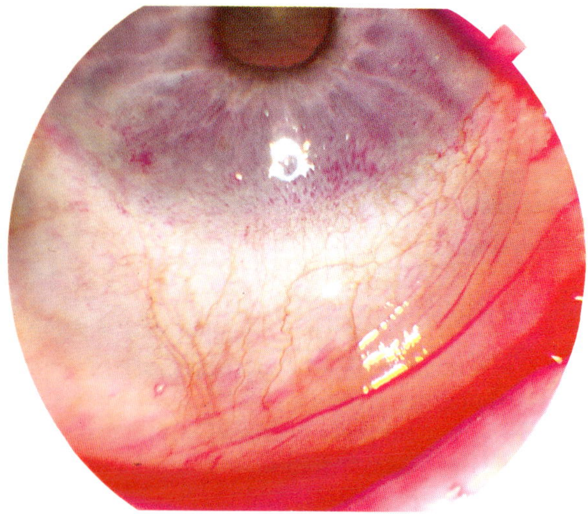

Fig. 4.3a Dry eye (stained Rose bengal)

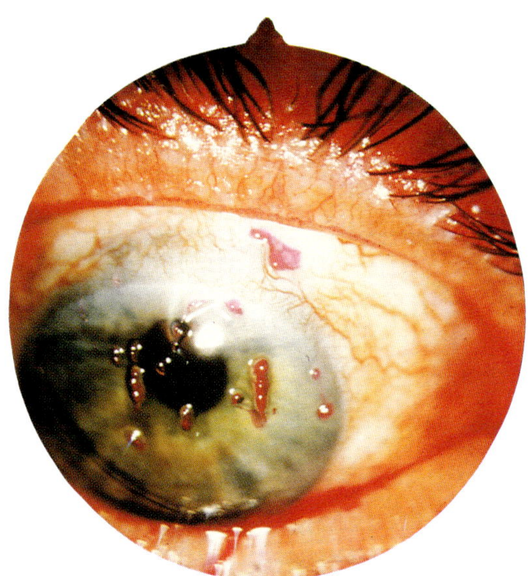

Fig. 4.3b Dry eye

lid and removed after 5 min. The length of the strip wetted is measured: 15 mm or more represents normal tear production.

Rose bengal staining (obtainable in Minims®) of the cornea and conjunctiva is another method of assessing the adequacy of tear secretion. Dry eyes show multiple punctate epithelial defects when examined under magnification. Mucous filaments may be seen adherent to the cornea (filamentary keratitis) (Figs 4.3a and b).

Although defective tear production cannot be cured, symptomatic relief can be obtained by the use of artificial tear supplements. Frequency of use varies with the degree of symptoms.

Patients whose dry eyes cause distress in spite of the use of artificial tears may be helped by surgical occlusion of the lacrimal puncta to conserve tears.

Dry eye problems which do not respond to simple measures should be referred for specialist assessment.

5. Conjunctiva and sclera

ANATOMY

The conjunctiva covers the anterior part of the eyeball and lines the lids. Its numerous glands moisten the surface. Lubrication is also provided by the lacrimal gland. Tears contain lysozyme, which inhibits the growth of organisms.

Deep to the conjunctiva is the sclera; the episclera is the layer between.

CONJUNCTIVA

Lacerations

Conjunctival wounds need to be treated with respect, for there may be a concealed injury to the eyeball. Visual acuity must be checked.

Conjunctiva heals rapidly if the wound edges are in apposition. Gaping wounds should be repaired.

If there is doubt about the integrity of the eye, refer.

Conjunctival foreign bodies

Foreign bodies blown into the eye, or loose lashes, commonly lodge in the lower fornix and are easily removed. If the foreign body is under the upper lid, not only does it scratch the cornea with each blink, but it cannot be removed without everting the lid.

The steps are as follows (Fig. 5.1):

1. The patient looks downwards with both eyes open.
2. The operator grasps the eyelashes between finger and thumb of one hand while, with the other, he presses the tip of a pencil, glass rod or an unfolded paper clip on the skin of the lid just above the tarsal plate.

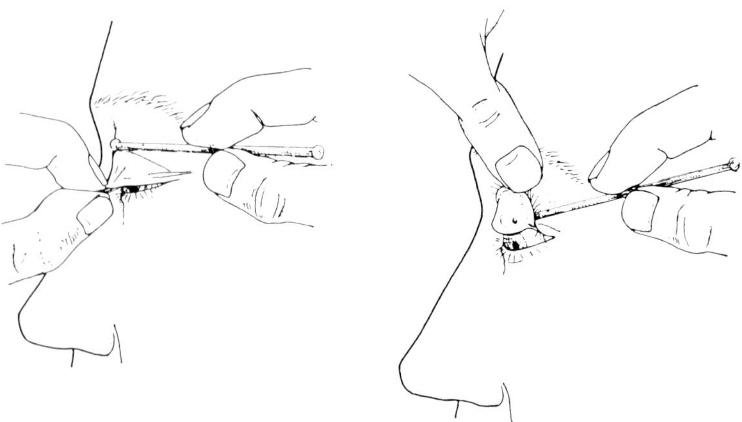

Fig. 5.1 Eversion of upper lid

3. The foreign body is removed.
4. Stain the cornea with fluorescein (p. 1). If an abrasion is found, antibiotic ointment should be used.

The upper and lower fornices of the conjunctiva are surprisingly capacious, and quite large foreign bodies may be concealed there.

Subconjunctival haemorrhage (Fig. 5.2)

A localized haemorrhage may follow injury to the eye and often is part of an orbital haematoma. The blood is absorbed in a week or two, but, if severe, the condition should raise suspicion of more serious injury such as fracture of the orbital walls or penetrating injury of the globe.

Spontaneous subconjunctival haemorrhage, often recurrent, is common in the elderly.

Chemical injuries of the conjunctiva

Energetic first aid may be critical after exposure to corrosive chemicals.

Workers in chemical industries or laboratories may receive splashes of liquid acids or alkalis in the eye. Although reflex tear production dilutes the irritant, immediate irrigation of the eyes with abundant water may be a sight-saving measure. The injured person's head should be held under a tap, while companions help

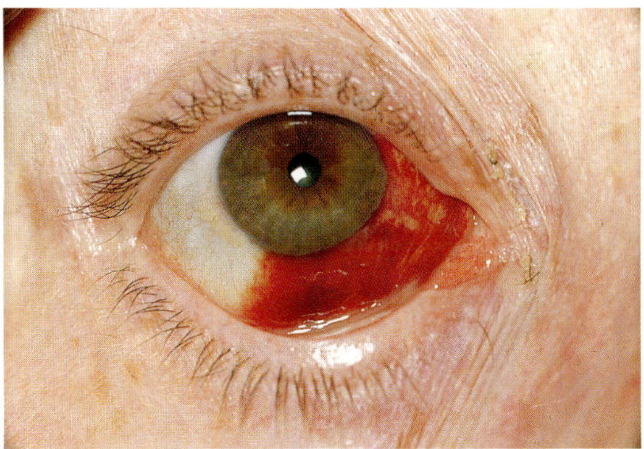

Fig. 5.2 Subconjunctival haemorrhage

to hold the eyes open while water runs over them. The subsequent management depends on the severity of the burning and the nature of the chemical concerned. Alkalis are, in general, more dangerous than acids. Liquid ammonia and caustic soda cause permanent corneal and conjunctival damage and possibly blindness. Any severe case should be referred after immediate first aid.

Lime requires special mention. Lime particles may be splashed in the face, especially in building workers, through powder flying up in mixing of cement. There is immediate blepharospasm and lacrimation, making examination difficult.

Treatment is as follows:

1. Anaesthetize with 1% amethocaine or 0.4% oxybuprocaine (Benoxinate®).
2. Remove all solid particles of lime from the conjunctiva, using forceps or cotton wool swabs.
3. Irrigate the eye thoroughly with water.
4. Stain with fluorescein.
5. If the cornea is clear and there is no conjunctival necrosis, instil antibiotic ointment.
6. If necrosis is present or the cornea hazy, refer.

Conjunctivitis (Fig. 5.3)

Inflammation of the conjunctiva is the commonest ophthalmic problem for the general practitioner. Symptoms are discomfort, dis-

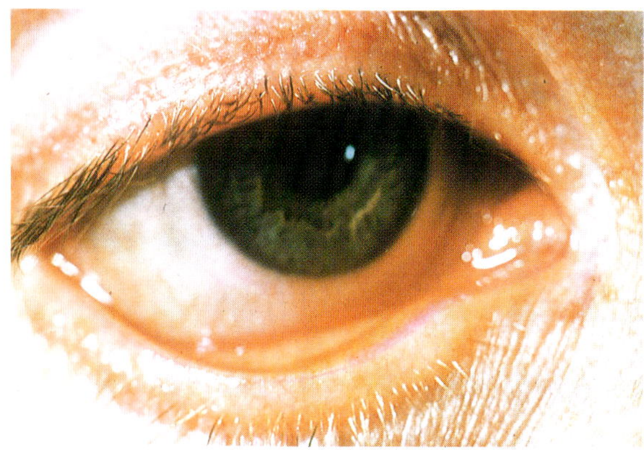

Fig. 5.3 Acute conjunctivitis

charge, and difficulty in opening the eye on waking (Tables 5.1 and 5.2). Signs are redness and discharge adherent to the lashes. Hypertrophy of lymphoid follicles may be seen, particularly in the lower fornix where they appear as shiny round swellings. The upper lid should be everted in the search for enlarged papillae on its conjunctival surface. Preauricular lymph node enlargement may be present. Visual acuity is not affected unless there is also corneal involvement, but the cornea should be stained with fluorescein and examined with magnification in a good light (see p. 1) to ensure that the epithelium is intact.

Some cases of chronic conjunctivitis defy definitive diagnosis and therapy. Such patients may be referred for assessment by an ophthalmologist.

Bacterial conjunctivitis

Purulent discharge and difficulty opening the eyes on waking are the cardinal features, with relatively mild, gritty discomfort. It is helpful to take a bacterial culture before starting treatment. Antibiotic drops — usually chloramphenicol or neomycin — should be given for at least 5 days; ointment may be given at night, in addition. A new sustained-release formulation of fusidic acid, Fucithalmic® viscous eye drops, dispensed from a tube, like ointment, have been shown in clinical trials to be of equal efficacy to chloramphenicol, and it enables a twice-daily dosage to be employed.

Table 5.1 Causes of conjunctivitis

Cause	Clinical features
Bacterial infections (see Table 5.2)	Mucopurulent discharge, crusting on lashes
Viral infection	Non-purulent. ± lower fornix follicles ± corneal lesions No response to antibiotics
Allergy	Marked in pollen season
Atopic conjunctivitis	History of allergy Itching the main symptom
Vernal conjunctivitis	Papillac — upper tarsal conjunctiva ± corneal lesions
Chemical and drug reactions	History of exposure ± lower fornix follicles
Mechanical causes	Eyelid abnormalities Trichiasis Exposure
Dry eye	Rose bengal staining. Reduced tear secretion ± associated systemic disorder

Table 5.2 Bacteria commonly causing conjunctivitis

Haemophilus influenzae
Streptococcus pneumoniae
Moraxella lacunata
Staphylococcus aureus

Chlamydial conjunctivitis (Fig. 5.4)

Bacteria of the genus *Chlamydia* live only within cells, forming intracellular inclusion bodies. *Chlamydia trachomatis* affects the human eye and genital tract. Following an acute initial infection, a chronic, often subclinical, phase follows.

Three distinct clinical syndromes are produced by infection of the conjunctiva by *C. trachomatis*:

1. *Neonatal inclusion conjunctivitis* (see p. 40).

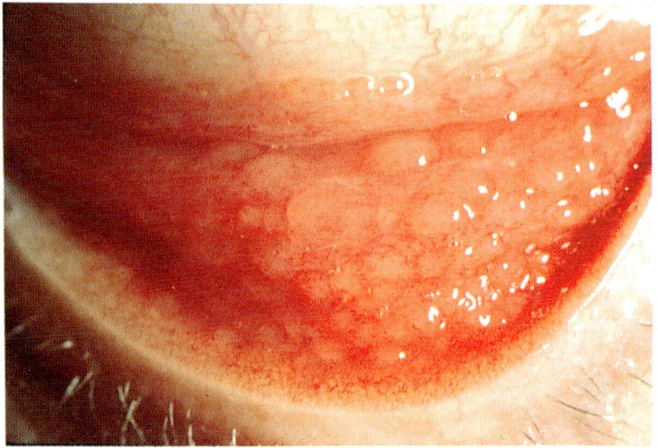

Fig. 5.4 Chlamydial conjunctivitis: follicles in lower fornix

2. *Endemic trachoma* — a chronic infection seen amongst underprivileged people living in warm dry climates with poor standards of hygiene. It is the world's major blinding condition. Sporadic cases seen in developed countries are usually inactive.

3. *C. trachomatis conjunctivitis* (adult inclusion conjunctivitis) is caused by strains of this organism which infect the genital tract and are transmitted to the eye following sexual contact. Sexually active adults are affected and the resultant conjunctivitis is florid, predominantly in the lower fornix, with follicle formation and punctate staining of the cornea.

The *diagnosis* is usually made after the condition has failed to respond to first-line treatment for bacterial conjunctivitis. Confirmation may be obtained by fluorescent microscopy of conjunctival cells for inclusion bodies. A swab is smeared on to a clean microscope slide and fixed with acetone or similar fixative. This method has the advantage that viable tissue is not required and it has replaced chlamydial culture in most centres.

Treatment. A 3-week course of 1% tetracycline ointment, with oral erythromycin 250 mg four times a day, is usually sufficient to eliminate both the conjunctival and genital infection. Inquiry should be made about sexual contacts and these should be treated by the general practitioner or venereologist.

Conjunctivitis in the newborn (ophthalmia neonatorum)

This is a notifiable disease and includes any purulent discharge from the eyes within 21 days of birth.

Table 5.3 Pathogens found in neonatal conjunctivitis

Pathogen	Recommended first antibiotic
N. gonorrhoeae	Oc. chloramphenicol
Staph. aureus	until sensitivities are known
Strep. pneumoniae	Oc. tetracycline for baby.
Haemophilus spp.	Tabs. erythromycin for mother
Chlamydia trachomatis	

Infection occurs during birth and appears within 2 or 3 days as gross oedema of the lids, between which pus escapes when an attempt is made to open the eye. The conjunctiva is congested and swollen (chemosis). The organisms commonly found on culture are listed in Table 5.3.

A culture should be taken from any newborn infant with conjunctivitis and the eyes should be examined to determine the state of the cornea. Treatment with chloramphenicol six times daily usually clears the infection. If there is any question of corneal damage, or the infection persists, viral cultures should also be taken and an attempt made to identify *Chlamydia*. Discharge must be removed as it forms. Treatment is best carried out in hospital.

Viral conjunctivitis

Adenovirus. Typically occurring in epidemics, eye infection by adenovirus is a potentially serious, bilateral disease. There is non-purulent, watery discharge. The conjunctivitis is associated with fine, punctate corneal ulcers and subepithelial opacities and, frequently, preauricular lymph node enlargement. The diagnosis can be confirmed by culture using a viral transport medium. The symptoms may persist for months or years with episodes of recurrence.

Strict hygienic precautions must be observed to minimize the risk of transfer of infection, especially at school and within the family.

Treatment is of little value, though symptomatic relief may be obtained from agents containing vasoconstrictors such as Otrivine-Antistin® drops. Patients in whom corneal complications are suspected should be referred for specialist care.

Herpes simplex. Primary herpes simplex infection may cause a short-lived conjunctivitis. Herpes simplex keratitis is discussed on page 55.

Herpes zoster. The affected eye may show marked conjunctival involvement. Management is discussed on page 56.

Other viral infections. Transient non-purulent conjunctivitis is a feature of many systemic viral infections. No specific treatment is required, the watering and redness settling with the resolution of the illness.

It is important to check the eyelid skin for previously unrecognized lesions of molluscum contagiosum (see p. 22) which may be the cause of recurrent conjunctivitis which defies treatment with antibiotics.

Allergic conjunctivitis

Allergic conjunctivitis occurs in several distinct forms:

1. *Acute allergic conjunctivitis.* This bilateral condition is an urticarial reaction to allergen reaching the conjunctiva directly. It may appear with dramatic suddenness and subside equally quickly. Treatment, apart from identifying and, if possible, avoiding the cause, is with topical and systemic antihistamines. Otrivine-Antistin® or Vasocon-A® drops, instilled every hour or two until the swelling subsides, usually prove satisfactory. Potentiation of acute, angle-closure glaucoma is a possible side-effect of these drugs.
2. *Chronic allergic conjunctivitis.* Usually a mild, bilateral inflammation with marked itching and no discharge; follicles may be present, particularly in the lower conjunctival fornices. The condition is most evident during the hay fever season. Typically, the cornea is not involved, but distinction must be made from drug-induced allergic conjunctivitis where contact lens soaking and cleaning solutions are the cause (p. 118).

Treatment should, where possible, be topical, and the condition can usually be satisfactorily managed in general practice.

Sodium cromoglycate (Opticrom®) drops 4 times daily are often effective. Alternatively, a topical antihistamine such as Otrivine-Antistin® or Vasocon-A® may help. Severe cases may require topical steroid drops, among which the preparations least likely to produce a marked rise of intraocular pressure — clobetasone (Eumovate®) and fluorometholone — are preferable. As with any other use of topical steroids, it is mandatory that the prescribing doctor checks the cornea for dendritic ulceration by staining with fluorescein before starting treatment. If treatment is continued for more than 4 weeks, checking of intraocular pressure by accurate tonometry is mandatory.

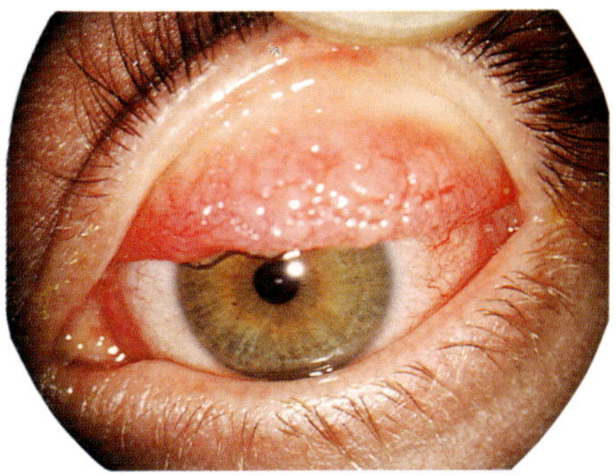

Fig. 5.5 Spring catarrh

Oral antihistamines such as terfenadine (Triludan®) 60 mg twice daily during active phases may also be helpful. A search for causative antigens by skin testing may help the patient, but desensitizing injections are generally not recommended except for life-threatening conditions such as asthma. A possible exception is seasonal hay fever, for which desensitization is of well-proven efficacy and the risks involved in its use may be considered justifiable.

3. *Vernal conjunctivitis* ('spring catarrh') (Fig. 5.5). Typically seen in atopic individuals in childhood and early adult life, the most serious of these IgE-mediated conditions is readily diagnosed by the finding of cobblestone-like papillae in the upper tarsal conjunctiva of both eyes on everting the upper lids. Numerous eosinophils are found on microscopic examination of the conjunctival scrapings. Corneal complications are common. Once diagnosed, the condition should be managed under specialist care, but the general practitioner may have to handle periodic exacerbations. Topical steroids such as prednisolone drops 0.5% or sodium cromoglycate (Opticrom®) are of about equal effectiveness. The condition usually resolves in early adult life, but permanent corneal scarring may remain.

4. *Drug-induced dermatoconjunctivitis* (see p. 118).

Chronic non-specific conjunctivitis

Conjunctivitis which persists despite treatment is common, though seldom disabling. Abnormalities of the eyelids — ectropion and entropion — and trichiasis should be excluded and tear secretion measured by Schirmer's test (p. 31). Referral to an ophthalmologist seldom results in a curative prescription, but useful reassurance may be obtained.

Degenerative conditions of the conjunctiva

Pinguecula (Fig. 5.6)

This is a common condition in adults of all ages. Near the corneoscleral junction medially and laterally, areas of subconjunctival degeneration occur, seen as creamy triangular plaques which may be elevated. Occasionally pingueculae become inflamed. Steroid drops remove the redness, but the usual precautions of staining the cornea to exclude ulceration, and avoidance of prolonged use of the drops, must be observed.

Pterygium (Fig. 5.7)

A wing-like area of subconjunctival degeneration occurs at the limbus and extends over the cornea. An opaque zone preceding the tip of the advancing pterygium indicates activity. If it is considered unsightly or threatens to cover the pupil, the patient should be referred for excision of the pterygium. A few days of considerable discomfort usually follow excision and recurrence is possible. The patient should be warned of this.

Tumours of the conjunctiva

These are rare and include the following:

Benign

Papillomata and *cysts* may be simply excised if causing discomfort or cosmetic blemish.

Naevus

Often close to the limbus, a conjunctival mole may be of any colour from coffee to jet black. It is slightly raised and has a nodular surface. Some become larger and darker at puberty. Unless excision is demanded for cosmetic reasons, no treatment is indicated. Any increase in size or vascularity of the lesion — like melanomata else-

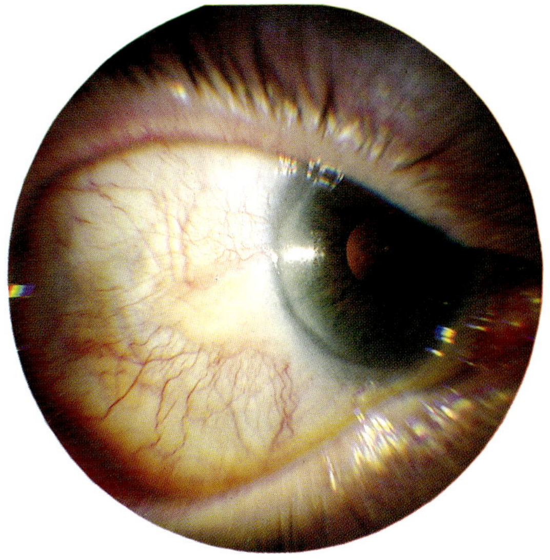

Fig. 5.6 Pinguecula

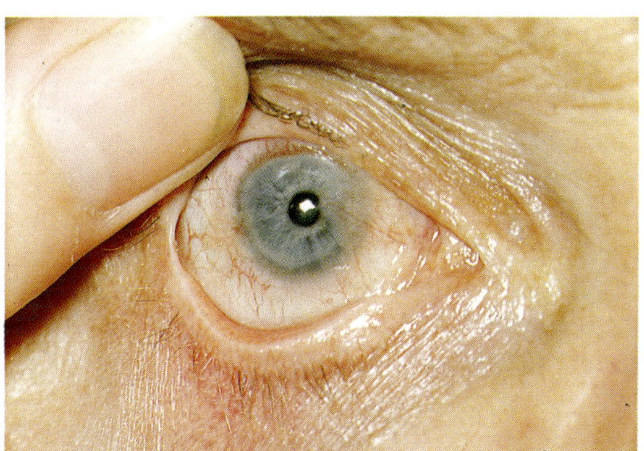

Fig. 5.7 Pterygium

where — should be regarded with suspicion. Malignant change occurs rarely and is an indication for wide excision.

Malignant

Carcinoma: very rare. *Malignant melanoma*: see above.

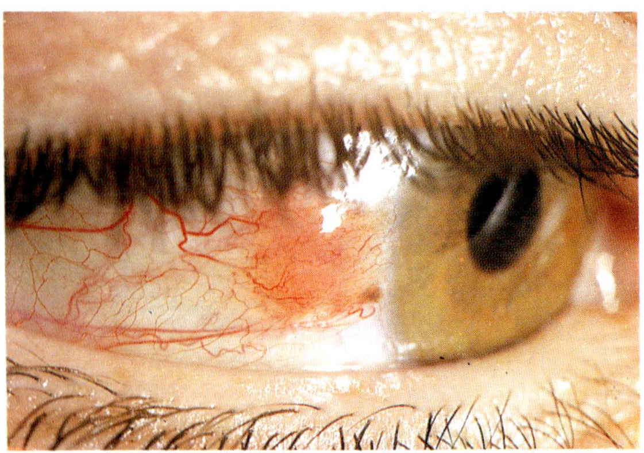

Fig. 5.8 Nodular episcleritis

EPISCLERA

Episcleritis (Fig. 5.8)

Inflammation of the episcleral tissue deep to the conjunctiva is usually unilateral, with slight discomfort and no discharge. The eye may be diffusely red or the inflammation localized; there may be an inflamed nodule, usually in the interpalpebral zone. The adjacent conjunctiva is not inflamed.

Although episcleritis may be associated with systemic disorders, it usually occurs for no known reason in healthy individuals and resolves spontaneously in a few weeks. Treatment with steroid drops such as prednisolone 0.5% four times daily is helpful. It is important to ensure that the cornea does not stain with fluorescein before starting treatment with steroids.

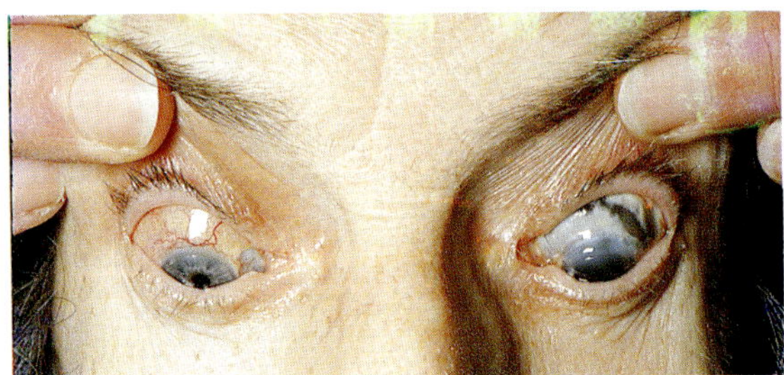

Fig. 5.9 Scleritis

Scleritis (Fig. 5.9)

Inflammation of the sclera is painful and often affects both eyes. The deeper vessels are engorged. Prolonged scleritis leads to scleral thinning so that the blue of the underlying ciliary body is seen. There may be associated sclerosis of the adjacent cornea, leading to opacification and marginal corneal thinning. Scleritis is usually seen in association with systemic disease — commonly rheumatoid arthritis complicated by vasculitis. The overall incidence of scleritis in rheumatoid patients is low and treatment is a matter for a specialist.

6. The cornea

ANATOMY

Despite its thinness (about 1 mm), the cornea is remarkably tough. The exposed surface is covered with epithelium continuous with that of the conjunctiva. Beneath the epithelium are numerous free nerve endings, explaining the sensitivity of the cornea and the pain resulting from injury or inflammation.

The cornea is bounded superficially by Bowman's membrane and, on its deep surface, by Descemet's membrane. The innermost layer is the endothelium, important in keeping the cornea optically clear by transfer of fluid from the stroma into the adjacent anterior chamber against the hydrostatic gradient of the intraocular pressure. The endothelium is of importance to the surgeon carrying out intraocular operations as its cells do not regenerate; they enlarge to cover a greater area as their number diminishes with age, in disease, or after trauma. If the endothelium fails, corneal oedema develops and vision is lost.

Peripherally, the cornea blends with the sclera at the limbus — a specialized region where most of the drainage of aqueous humour takes place. The inner aspect of this area contains the trabecular meshwork, communicating, via the canal of Schlemm, with the episcleral veins on the surface of the globe. This is the outflow pathway for the aqueous humour.

CONGENITAL AND HEREDITARY DISEASE

Keratoconus (conical cornea) (Fig. 6.1)

Having been normal in childhood, the cornea loses its normal curvature and becomes increasingly steeply curved, with resultant irregular refraction of the entering light. Visual acuity falls, usually during early adult life, and cannot be improved by spectacles. No

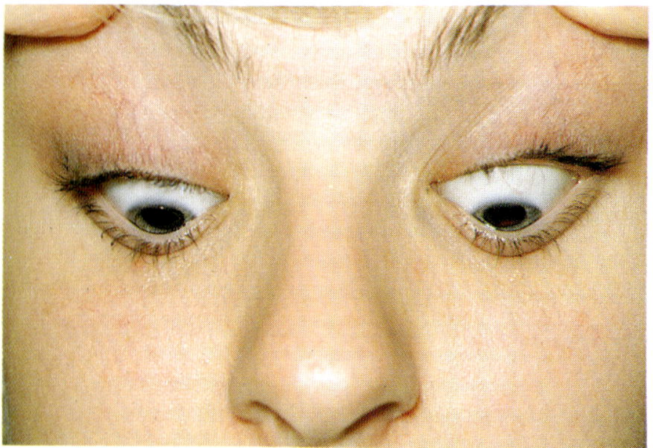

Fig. 6.1 Keratoconus (note contact lens on right eye)

medical treatment can arrest this process, but satisfactory vision can often be obtained with hard contact lenses (see p. 115). If corneal oedema or scarring develops, vision may be restored by corneal grafting. Keratoconus can most easily be demonstrated by observing the lower lid curvature when the patient looks down (Munson's sign).

Corneal dystrophies

An obscure group of conditions occurring more commonly in adult life and with a familial tendency. Corneal opacities develop bilaterally and interfere increasingly with vision. Both eyes are affected. There are no inflammatory signs, except in rare superficial dystrophies in which there is recurrent corneal erosion. The pathological process cannot be reversed by medical treatment, but corneal grafting usually gives improvement.

Fuchs' dystrophy is of particular importance in the elderly. It is a degenerative condition which affects the endothelium, with a tendency to corneal oedema when the endothelial cells are no longer able to maintain corneal clarity. When associated with cataract, Fuchs' dystrophy presents a difficult problem for the surgeon, who is faced with the need to carry out both cataract extraction and full-thickness corneal grafting. Fuchs' dystrophy may recur after grafting.

Congenital limbal dermoid

This congenital, non-progressive tumour occurs at the corneal margin and covers a variable extent of the cornea. It is pearly white, elevated, and may have hairs on its surface. Excision is often required on cosmetic grounds, though a permanent scar remains.

TRAUMA

Corneal abrasion

This is an injury involving the epithelium. There is pain, lacrimation, photophobia and blepharospasm. The diagnosis is confirmed by staining the cornea with fluorescein (Fig. 6.2). Examination is easier if the eye is anaesthetized with a drop of local anaesthetic, and, if there is a possibility of a foreign body, a thorough search of the conjunctival sac, with eversion of the upper lid (see p. 35) is necessary. Treatment is with antibiotic ointment and a firmly applied pad until the epithelial defect has healed — normally within 24–48 hours. Infection and failure to heal will lead to corneal ulceration.

Recurrent corneal erosion

Apparently trivial corneal injuries may lead to intermittent recurrence of symptoms. A mother whose eye is injured by her baby's finger is typical. Following healing of the initial abrasion, the

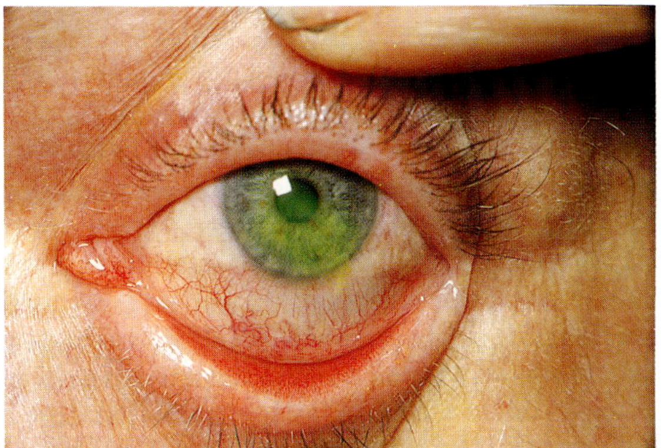

Fig. 6.2 Corneal abrasion

patient wakes from sleep with pain because an area of unstable epithelium has been shed on first opening the eye. Symptoms subside during the day, as adjacent epithelial cells slide over to cover the defect. This sequence is repeated at intervals.

Plentiful application of a non-steroid ointment at night for a month or two is usually effective: Lacri-Lube® ointment, obtainable without prescription, is suitable. Alternative treatments involve removal of the affected area of epithelium with alcohol, after anaesthetizing the cornea, or the use of a soft, 'bandage' contact lens for an extended period. Difficult cases should be referred for confirmation of the diagnosis by slit lamp examination, and for specialist advice about management.

Welder's flash ('arc eye')

Welder's flash and snow blindness are similar conditions and are due to exposure to ultraviolet light. After an interval of 6 or 8 h, intense bilateral lacrimation, blepharospasm and photophobia develop.

Examination may not be possible until the eyes have been anaesthetized with 1% amethocaine. Once the blepharospasm has been relieved, multiple punctate corneal erosions are seen to stain with fluorescein. The lesions heal within a few hours. Local anaesthetic drops and reassurance are the only treatment required.

Foreign bodies

Usually there is a clear history of the entry of the foreign body, though other irritants, such as a loose lash or a subtarsal foreign body, cause similar symptoms. A good light and magnification help with removal. A drop of local anaesthetic such as 1% amethocaine is instilled and the foreign body removed. If it is loosely adherent to the cornea it may be removed with a cotton wool 'bud' or the corner of a tissue. A sterile 17-gauge needle is a convenient instrument to pick a foreign body off the cornea. Antibiotic ointment is used four times a day for 4 days and the patient reports back if the eye is uncomfortable or the vision blurred. Mydriatics are usually unnecessary: atropine, with its prolonged action, is never required. Following the removal of a metallic foreign body, a rust ring may remain; this is more readily removed after 2 or 3 days use of antibiotic ointment.

Patients should be advised about protective measures.

Perforations of the cornea

All perforations, and cases in which there is suspicion, should be referred, and the patient instructed to take nothing by mouth in order to be ready for general anaesthesia. *Normal visual acuity is not inconsistent with the presence of an intraocular foreign body.* A history of hammering metal on metal, with no evident superficial foreign body, suggests an intraocular metallic fragment, and the finding of a subconjunctival haemorrhage heightens suspicion. X-ray of the eye usually demonstrates a metallic foreign body, however small.

Laceration of the cornea causes reduction in depth of the anterior chamber as compared with the other eye, or distortion of the pupil. Injury to deeper structures may be seen as lens opacities or haemorrhage in the eye (see p. 103).

Early detection is of great importance in successful management. Damage to the eye by a retained intraocular foreign body, by infection, or by resulting retinal detachment, may be irreversible. 'Missed' intraocular foreign bodies are an unfortunate but regular cause of justified medicolegal claims. If there is any suspicion of penetration, refer to hospital.

CORNEAL INFLAMMATION (Keratitis)

A corneal ulcer is usually painful. There may have been previous episodes of corneal ulceration or other eye disease, or a history of a foreign body or trauma. If contact lenses are worn, they should be suspected as the cause of any keratitis.

Visual acuity is reduced if the central cornea is involved. Fluorescein staining and inspection in good light will show the size, situation and shape of any ulcer.

Causes of corneal ulceration

The cause may be bacterial, fungal, a foreign body, viral, exposure or toxic reaction.

Bacterial keratitis

Infection usually enters the cornea after injury. The eye is painful, photophobic and watery. There is a sensation of something in the eye due to movement of the lids over the epithelial defect.

The eye is red, most markedly in the quadrant where the ulcer lies. Visual acuity is usually reduced. A greyish area of oedema and opacity may be seen before stain is used. Fluorescein demarcates the edges of the ulcer. A search should be made for a foreign body on the cornea, or under the upper lid.

Before starting treatment it is important to identify the causative organism. This involves taking cultures and a direct scraping from the ulcer bed for urgent microscopic examination. These cases should be referred.

Treatment

Intensive topical antibiotic applications are needed, usually combined with a mydriatic such as atropine 1%. Hospital admission may be desirable. Padding the eye is usually unnecessary.

Failure to heal within 48 h or so, or the development of a level of pus — a hypopyon — within the anterior chamber, are indications for urgent referral.

Marginal keratitis (Fig. 6.3)

This represents a local hypersensitivity reaction to conjunctival infection by certain organisms — usually *Staphylococcus aureus*. Conjunctivitis may be slight, but there is photophobia, pain and vascular congestion at the limbus, where round or elongated ulcers, or subepithelial corneal infiltrates, are found. These do not progress centrally. In addition to treating the conjunctivitis with antibiotic

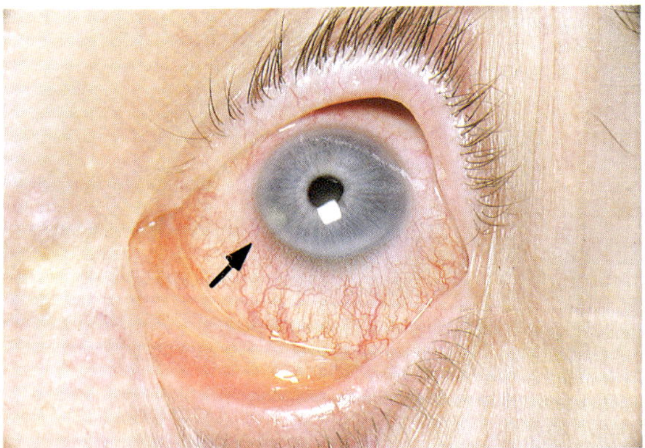

Fig. 6.3 Marginal corneal ulcer

drops or ointment, a topical steroid may be used. This is one of the few ophthalmic situations where the use of combined antibiotic–steroid is justified over a short time, provided that no dendritic ulcer (q.v.) is present.

Viral keratitis

Herpes simplex keratitis (dendritic ulcer)

This infection is primarily confined to the corneal epithelium, and the resultant dendritic ulcer is a common and serious condition. It presents as an irritable eye (often without much discomfort) and is diagnosed after fluorescein staining (Fig. 6.4) as a branching ulcer. The virus lies dormant in the trigeminal nerve between attacks.

Treatment is with a topical antiviral. Of several available, the most effective and least toxic is acyclovir (Zovirax®) ointment, used five times daily until the ulcer has healed. This should be under specialist supervision, but initial treatment may be started by the general practitioner as soon as the diagnosis is made.

Recurrence is common, and is treated in the same way. Steroid preparations should never be used in general practice if herpes simplex infection is suspected.

Complications. Amoeboid ulceration is a more advanced form of the disease in which the ulcer spreads to assume a confluent pattern. Treatment is with antiviral agents.

Disciform keratitis and kerato-uveitis. Herpes simplex infection of the deeper layers of the cornea leads to central corneal thickening

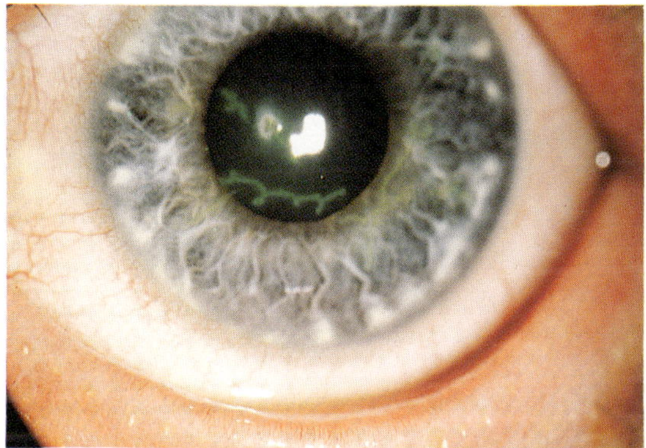

Fig. 6.4 Dendritic ulcer

and opacification described as 'disciform keratitis'. There is usually associated uveitis. Treatment is difficult and needs to be carefully monitored in a specialist unit; frequently, diluted steroid drops are used at the same time as an antiviral agent. Activity may last for months. Permanent scarring of the cornea is common and may necessitate corneal grafting.

Fortunately, herpes simplex keratitis is usually unilateral.

Herpes zoster (Fig. 6.5)

Corneal ulceration may occur during the acute stage of ophthalmic herpes zoster; conjunctival inflammation, uveitis and secondary glaucoma are also seen, as is a dendritic-like ulcer. Vesicles on the nose suggest eye involvement. Later, corneal sensation may be impaired and lid deformities occur, resulting in a chronic keratitis which is difficult to manage.

Treatment. This is controversial and may be difficult. The patient may be ill and unwilling to attend an eye clinic.

On first appearance of the skin eruption, oral acyclovir has proven efficacy. Acyclovir (Zovirax®) 800 mg tablets are given 4-hourly, omitting the night-time dose, for 7 days. Adequate hydration must be maintained, particularly in the elderly. This expensive treatment

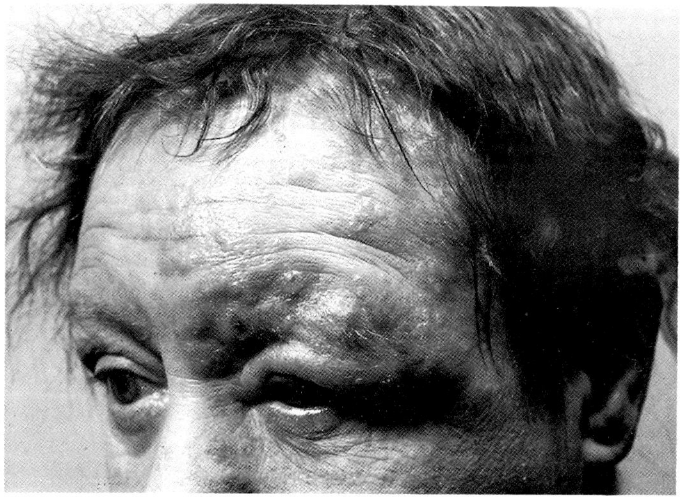

Fig. 6.5 Ophthalmic herpes zoster

is of doubtful value if started more than 24 h after the onset of the skin eruption.

There is no general agreement as to what to apply to the affected skin; it is probably best to put on nothing at all — the infection is in the nerves, not the skin. Petroleum jelly relieves itching; 5% acyclovir (Zovirax®) cream is available but its superiority has not been proved.

Topical treatment to the eye should consist of acyclovir (Zovirax®) five times daily for 5 days or until the eye is white. If it is suspected that the eye is involved, the patient should be referred, but it is important to start treatment at the earliest time possible.

It may be difficult to open the lids, but a relative or nurse should be able to get some ointment into the conjunctival sac.

Swelling of the subcutaneous tissues around the other eye is not a cause for concern. This is usually tissue fluid which tracks across the midline in a patient who lies in bed with the affected side uppermost.

General measures. Analgesics will generally be required: co-praxamol (Distalgesic®), DF118® and buprenorphine (Temgesic®) (200–400 mg 6–8 hourly) are all suitable. The H_2 receptor antagonist, cimetidine, 400 mg twice daily by mouth, has been advocated, as has amantadine (Symmetrel®), 100 mg twice daily for 5 days, but their effectiveness has not been proved conclusively by clinical trial. Systemic prednisolone, 80 mg daily, reducing over 1 week, is recommended for patients with neurological complications (see below).

Complications, apart from eye and lid inflammation and their direct sequelae, include extraocular muscle paralysis, most commonly involving the third nerve, optic neuritis and hemiparesis. Postherpetic neuralgia may be a long-term problem. Herpes zoster in patients with impaired immunity, either from disease or from the use of immunosuppressive drugs, is likely to be more prolonged and severe; hospital admission is essential. Hospital admission should also be considered for any patient in whom the eye is involved.

Adenoviral keratitis

This epidemic condition is discussed under conjunctival infections (p. 41).

Fungal keratitis

Injuries, particularly by vegetable matter, occasionally cause corneal ulcers which are resistant to conventional antibiotic treatment. Necrotic material seen in the ulcer bed may prove to contain fungi.

In common with other corneal ulcers which fail to respond to antibiotics, referral is essential.

Other forms of keratitis

Acanthamoeba keratitis

Acanthamoeba is a protozoon commonly found in soil and water. It may infect the cornea — contact lens wearers are most at risk, accounting for 80% of cases. Poor hygiene practices, notably the preparation, at home, of non-sterile saline solutions and the rinsing of contact lenses with tap water, are important sources of infection.

The infection produces severe, painful ulceration of the cornea, which is refractory to antibiotics. The organism can be demonstrated by microscopy and culture. The most effective treatment is with Brolene® drops. Diagnosis and management are a matter for the specialist.

Keratoconjunctivitis sicca

The triad of dry eyes, dry mouth and collagen disease particularly affects patients with rheumatoid arthritis. The symptoms are discomfort and, sometimes, mucoid discharge, occasionally progressing to frank corneal ulceration with severe pain. Mucus filaments may be seen adherent to the cornea (filamentary keratitis). Staining the dry eye with rose bengal (obtainable in solution as Minims®) shows multiple small red dots on cornea and conjunctiva, representing epithelial defects (Figs 4.3a and b). Defective tear production may be confirmed by Schirmer's test (see p. 31), though dry eyes are common in older people without systemic disease.

Treatment is with artificial tear supplements, of which a number of proprietary preparations are available without prescription. A patient may be advised to try several and to persist with that which is found most acceptable. The drops should be used for symptomatic relief as often as needed. Dry eye is a variable condition and the need for drops will change according to the patient's state as well as the prevailing weather conditions. Dry environments such as centrally heated houses with inadequate humidification, and cars with the heaters blowing hot air, are particularly troublesome.

Severe cases should be referred for assessment by an ophthalmologist. Surgical occlusion of the lacrimal puncta may be a useful additional measure, and mucolytic drops such as acetylcysteine 5% (Ilube®) may also be recommended.

Other rheumatoid conditions. Any rheumatoid patient with painful eyes not responding to artificial tear supplements should be referred for slit lamp examination of the eye and further assessment.

Neuroparalytic keratitis

Loss of corneal sensation deprives the cornea of one of its protective mechanisms and may be followed by ulceration. In addition to herpes zoster affecting the ophthalmic division (see p. 56) any lesion of the fifth nerve which produces corneal anaesthesia may lead to keratitis. Protection of the cornea, by the copious use of ointment at night and spectacles with protective side pieces, may be sufficient. Patients at risk of corneal ulceration should be referred: tarsorrhaphy (temporary or permanent partial closure of the lids), or 'bandage' soft contact lenses may be required.

Rosacea keratitis (Fig. 6.6)

Rosacea leads to reddening of the skin of the face, telangiectasia and episodes of inflammation. The cause is unknown. Possible ophthalmic complications are blepharitis, chalazia, conjunctivitis and keratitis.

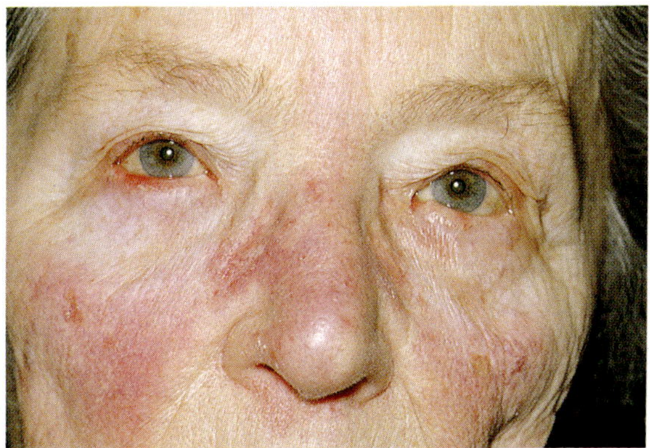

Fig. 6.6 Rosacea

Corneal involvement begins with marginal vascular infiltration; ulceration and opacification may follow. Treatment with low dosage oral tetracycline (250 mg b.d.) for at least 2 months usually controls exacerbations.

Bell's palsy

Idiopathic facial palsy may lead to exposure keratitis. While waiting for recovery of movement, the patient should be supplied with plenty of antibiotic ointment to put in the affected eye at night. Taping the lids together at night is often helpful.

Dysthyroid exophthalmos

Proptosis due to this or any other cause may place the cornea at risk from exposure. Dysthyroid eye disease is considered on page 155. Plenty of ointment at night is the first measure, reinforced, if necessary, by taping the lids (see above).

Other causes of exposure keratitis

Any debilitating disease may lead to the patient sleeping with imperfectly closed eyes, with consequent drying of the cornea, seen as a lack of normal lustre in the epithelium. Ointment should be instilled regularly. In severe cases, padding of the eyes with a paraffin gauze square under the pad may be necessary until normal lid closure returns.

DEGENERATIVE CONDITIONS OF THE CORNEA

Band-shaped opacity

In some degenerate eyes and in those which have sustained previous injury or inflammation, a horizontal opacity develops in the interpalpebral portion of the cornea, with deposition of calcium in its superficial layers. Patients with this condition should be referred — treatment with chelating agents applied under local anaesthesia may be considered.

Pterygium (Fig. 5.7) (see Ch. 5)

A degenerative condition arising in the conjunctiva and extending horizontally as a wing-like opacity of the cornea. May need surgery.

MATERIAL FOR CORNEAL GRAFTING

The extension of organ transplantation to include kidney, liver, heart and lungs, and the problem of transmissible virus diseases, particularly hepatitis and AIDS, and also the slow virus diseases affecting the central nervous system, have made corneal grafting dependent on organ donor centres. Fortunately it is now possible to store donor cornea for extended periods, making corneal grafting a procedure which can be undertaken on a planned basis.

In the United Kingdom the service is centralized at The United Kingdom Transplant Service, Southmead Road, Bristol BS10 5ND, telephone 0272 507777, to whom enquiries should be directed.

7. The middle coat of the eye

ANATOMY

The vascular, pigmented middle coat of the eye — the uveal tract — is in three parts — iris, ciliary body and choroid. The iris diaphragm lies against the lens, separating the anterior and posterior chambers of the eye. The ciliary body produces aqueous humour and permits variation of focus of the eye (accommodation) through its attachment to the lens by the zonular fibres. The ciliary muscle is innervated by the parasympathetic component of the third cranial nerve.

The sphincter pupillae (parasympathetic, third nerve) and dilator pupillae (cervical sympathetic) control the size of the pupil. The highly vascular choroid and the central retinal artery together nourish the retina.

CONGENITAL ABNORMALITIES

Aniridia

Congenital absence of the iris is a rare, genetically determined abnormality. Affected individuals are likely to have poor vision and to develop glaucoma. Aniridia is part of a spectrum of uncommon disorders of the anterior segment of the eye, collectively known as mesodermal dysgenesis.

Albinism

Pigment is absent from the eye (ocular albinism) or from the whole body. Vision is poor and nystagmus occurs. Albinoid children should be referred for specialist assessment.

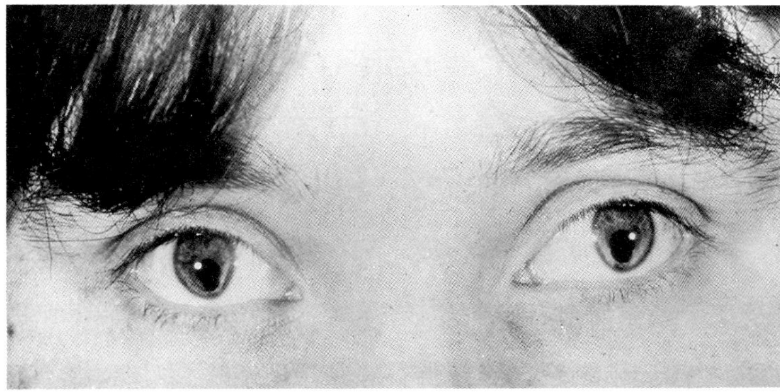

Fig. 7.1 Iris colobomata

Colobomata (Fig. 7.1)

Incomplete closure of the fetal choroidal fissure of the developing eye leaves a defect in the uveal tract in its lower nasal quadrant. Colobomata extending posteriorly in the choroid may be associated with poor vision.

TRAUMA

Non-perforating eye injuries due to squash balls, shuttlecocks, etc. small enough to enter the orbit may damage the uveal tissues.

Hyphaema (Fig. 10.1) (see Ch. 10)

Bleeding into the anterior chamber causes blurred vision. When the blood has settled, a level is seen in the anterior chamber. Patients with hyphaema are usually referred to hospital because of the possibility of secondary haemorrhage: though uncommon, this can be disastrous. Contusion severe enough to produce hyphaema frequently causes damage to the anterior chamber angle and may lead to glaucoma years later (p. 144).

If a patient with traumatic hyphaema cannot be admitted to hospital, bed rest should be advised until the blood has been absorbed.

Traumatic mydriasis

Paralysis of the iris sphincter following contusion may lead to a persistently dilated pupil; there may also be impairment of accommodation. Recovery after a few weeks is common.

Iridodialysis

A tear of the iris root.

Choroidal tear

Force from a contusion injury transmitted to the posterior segment of the eye may result in a crescentic tear of the choroid, usually temporal to the disc. Severe visual impairment may result; there is no treatment.

UVEAL INFLAMMATION

Suppurative inflammation of the uveal tract is usually obvious and requires urgent referral. *Non-suppurative* uveitis, an important cause of blindness, is more difficult to diagnose and remains poorly understood. Although occasionally secondary to other ocular disorders such as keratitis and cataract, most cases of uveitis are endogenous.

Acute anterior uveitis (iritis) (Fig. 7.2)

This is the form most important in general practice. Presenting as a red and photophobic eye, there is engorgement of the blood ves-

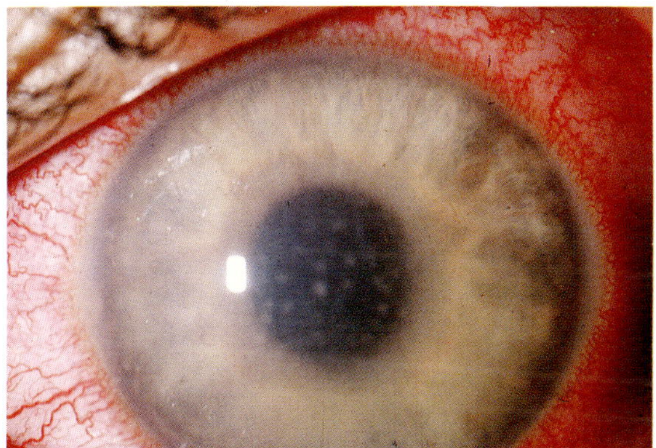

Fig. 7.2 Acute iritis

sels around the limbus; the pupil is small and may be irregular, adhering to the lens (posterior synechiae). Visual acuity is frequently impaired. Clumps of leucocytes adhering to the posterior surface of the cornea (keratic precipitates) may be seen under magnification. Keratic precipitates and posterior synechiae are diagnostic of uveitis. Exact diagnosis may be difficult. All suspected cases should be referred urgently.

The cause, in most cases, cannot be found, although about half have the HLA B27 antigen. Systemic disorders such as juvenile rheumatoid arthritis, sarcoidosis, ankylosing spondylitis and Reiter's disease may be found.

Treatment is with topical corticosteroids, with cyclopentolate 1% or atropine 1% to dilate the pupil. Steroids, either systemically or by injection round the eye, are required if drops fail to control the inflammation. Recurrences are common. A patient known previously to have uveitis who presents again to his general practitioner may be treated initially with steroid drops and a mydriatic, provided examination of the cornea (with fluorescein) has shown no dendritic ulcer to be present.

Posterior uveitis (choroiditis, chorioretinitis) (Fig. 7.3)

This condition is painless and the eye is usually white. Blurred vision or the finding of fundus lesions at routine ophthalmoscopy are the usual modes of presentation.

Most cases are of unknown cause and treatment is correspondingly haphazard and unrewarding. Systemic granulomatous conditions such as sarcoidosis, tuberculosis and syphilis are occasionally found.

Two specific forms of posterior uveitis deserve mention:

1. Toxoplasmosis

Either congenital or an acquired infection. The former is of significance in the eye, but the acquired disease, which may occur at any age, usually causes no symptoms.

Congenital toxoplasmosis (Fig. 7.4). The organism has a predilection for central nervous tissue and, in the extreme form, causes severe brain damage. Convulsions may be the first symptom, and intracranial calcification may be evident on X-ray examination of the skull. Ocular toxoplasmosis produces scarring in the retina and choroid — a white lesion surrounded by accumulated black

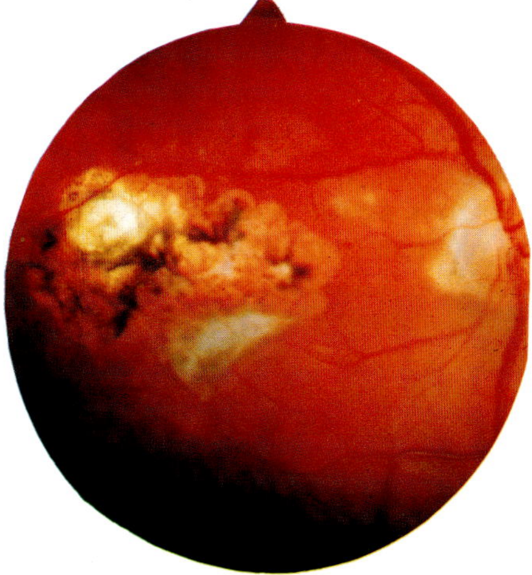

Fig. 7.3 Choroiditis in inactive congenital toxoplasmosis

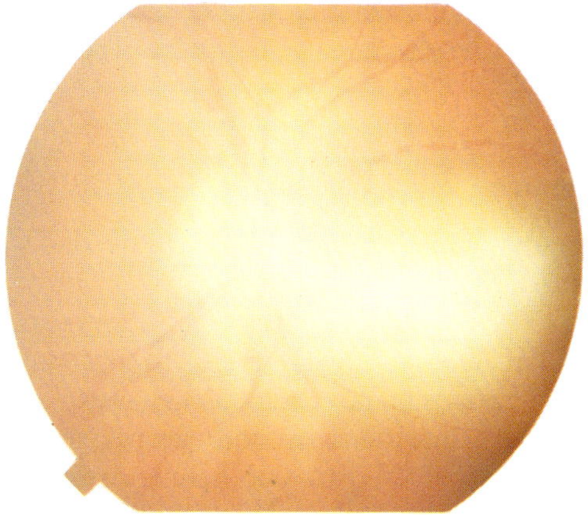

Fig. 7.4 Active juxtapapillary choroiditis

pigment in the inactive stage. Such a focus at the posterior pole prevents the development of macular vision.

Toxoplasmosis lesions in the eye may undergo apparently spontaneous reactivation, producing signs of posterior uveitis, often with associated inflammation in the anterior segment. Cloudiness of the vitreous causes blurred vision; visual loss is profound if the reactivated focus lies near the macula or optic disc (Fig. 7.4).

Diagnosis is usually made on clinical grounds, but antibody tests such as the toxoplasmosis dye titre may help.

Treatment is unnecessary unless vision is impaired, but any patient known to have ocular toxoplasmosis who notices blurred vision should be referred. Steroids by mouth or by intraorbital injection are usually combined with an antimicrobial agent such as clindamycin 300 mg four times weekly for some weeks. Pseudomembranous colitis is a rare but serious side effect of this drug.

2. Toxocariasis

Infection of the eye by the nematode worm *Toxocara canis* is an uncommon but serious form of posterior uveitis, usually occurring in young children who play in ground contaminated by the excrement of puppies which have not been 'wormed'. The parasite reaches the posterior pole of the eye, producing a choroidoretinal lesion which irreversibly destroys central vision. Fortunately, it is generally unilateral. Presentation usually results from routine visual acuity testing or the detection of a squint. Treatment has little to offer.

Acquired immune deficiency syndrome (AIDS)

AIDS is a multisystem disorder caused by infection with the human immunodeficiency virus (HIV), and involvement of most parts of the body has been recorded. The ocular adnexa may be involved by Kaposi's sarcoma. The uveal tract, vitreous and retina may all be affected by opportunistic infections associated with 'full-blown' AIDS, and severe infections by both herpes simplex and herpes zoster, with their characteristic ophthalmic manifestations, are not infrequently seen.

The commonest sign of AIDS in the eye, and that most likely to be found by the general practitioner, is the appearance of a number of 'cotton wool spots' in the retinae of both eyes. The mechanism by which these are produced is uncertain, but they are thought to be a sign of intravascular clotting. Cotton wool spots in the retina may appear in otherwise asymptomatic carriers of HIV infection (see Fig. 9.15).

Most dramatic are the haemorrhagic retinal lesions, described as 'cottage cheese and ketchup', due to retinal infection by cytomegalovirus. These may severely impair vision, but are unlikely to be encountered in general practice as they are a feature of the advanced stages of AIDS.

TUMOURS OF THE UVEAL TRACT

Iris

Tumours of the iris are rare, but any patient concerned that a tumour may be developing should be referred for a specialist opinion.

Ciliary body

Malignant melanoma occasionally develops in the ciliary body causing distortion of the pupil or detachment of the retina. These tumours, if not too large, may be treated by local resection with preservation of useful vision.

Choroid

Benign melanoma

Flat, pigmented areas usually occur in the posterior half of the fundus. They are seldom significantly elevated and there is no associated retinal detachment. Distinction between larger benign melanomas and malignant tumours may be difficult — cases of doubt should be referred for observation, serial fundus photography, and B-scan ultrasonography (see p. 162).

Malignant melanoma (Fig. 7.5)

These tumours arise anywhere in the uveal tract — iris, ciliary body or choroid. Iris melanomas must be distinguished from the commonly occurring benign naevi. They seldom grow aggressively but if malignancy is suspected the tumour should be excised with a segment of iris.

Malignant melanoma of the ciliary body and choroid is a life-threatening condition. The lesion is elevated and tends to cause an associated retinal detachment, with peripheral field loss and, later, impairment of central vision. Distant metastases are common and a search must be made for evidence of metastatic spread when planning treatment.

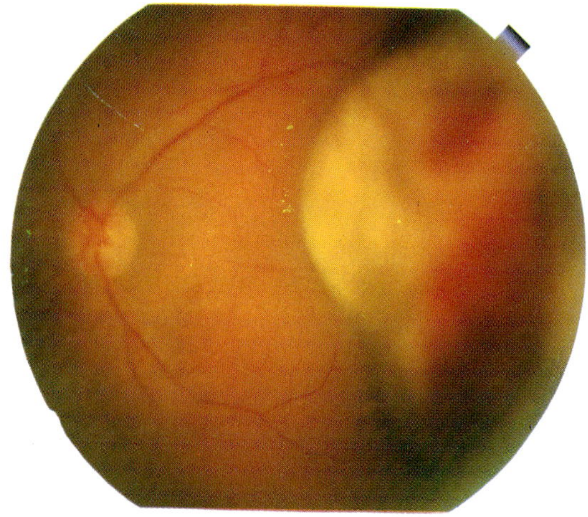

Fig. 7.5 Malignant melanoma

Treatment is controversial: patients treated by enucleation have been shown to be at greater risk of dying from metastases in the years immediately following surgery then those left untreated. Conversely, the prospect of extrascleral extension cannot be viewed with equanimity. Local resection of the tumour with preservation of the eye is sometimes feasible, as are various forms of radiation therapy. Patients over 70 are sometimes left untreated if the tumour is small.

Metastatic tumours

These tumours present similarly to malignant melanoma, but their growth is more rapid. Palliative radiation may be justified. Tumours arising from breast carcinoma usually respond to Tamoxifen®.

8. Cataract

Any opacity in the lens is a cataract. Many are either non-progressive or increase only slowly; only a small proportion eventually need surgical treatment. However, cataract is the commonest single reason for referral by general practitioners to ophthalmologists and its treatment forms the largest part of the surgical workload of most eye departments.

The general practitioner will be involved in deciding whom to refer with cataract and, perhaps, in discussion with the patient of the advice given. He may also participate in the postoperative management, particularly with regard to the recognition of posterior capsule opacification. An understanding of the issues involved is therefore essential.

CLASSIFICATION OF CATARACT

1. Congenital
2. Cataract associated with other disorders
   a. metabolic
   b. syndromes of multiple congenital deformity
   c. skin disease
   d. drugs
   e. physical causes: trauma, heat, ionizing radiation, electric shock
   f. secondary to other eye disease
3. Senile.

Congenital cataract

The lens is developed by the infolding of a vesicle from the surface ectoderm. Within this vesicle, layers of lens fibres are developed, the oldest being forced toward the centre and the youngest being

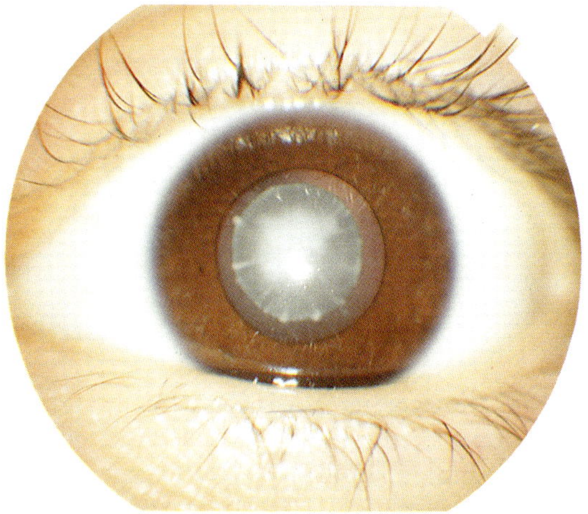

Fig. 8.1 Cataract

found on the surface. Interference with this process results in opacity. Rubella, for example, during the first trimester of pregnancy, conveys a definite risk of the child being born with congenital defects in the eye, ear or heart. Cataract due to rubella is a sporadic disorder; many congenital cataracts are familial.

Incomplete congenital cataracts are known as lamellar (zonular) cataracts. While the majority of congenital lens opacities do not increase after birth, some types, particularly of a punctate variety, become more dense in later life and may then require surgery (Fig. 8.1).

The presence of an opaque lens in the eye of an infant is an absolute indication for referral within the first few days of life if there is to be any prospect of useful treatment. Total removal of the cataractous lens, together with the anterior part of the vitreous — lensectomy — is usually the operation of choice. Optical correction can subsequently be provided by 'soft' contact lenses suitable for long-term wear. Close supervision is essential or amblyopia (p. 123) will negate the benefits of surgery. Retinal detachment, often many years after surgery for congenital cataract, is an important potential complication and must be taken into account when deciding whether to advise operation.

Cataract associated with other disorders

Metabolic

1. *Diabetes mellitus.* Diabetics develop cataract at an earlier age than non-diabetics, and cataract patients attending eye clinics are routinely examined for glycosuria. In one study 3% were found to have diabetes, previously undiagnosed. The management of cataract does not differ from that in non-diabetics, but postoperative complications are rather more common and removal of a dense cataract may reveal diabetic retinal changes.
2. *Galactosaemia.* Cataracts in newborn infants with galactosaemia are reversible by early treatment.
3. *Hypocalcaemia.* Cataract, characteristically of the subcapsular type, may follow hypocalcaemia from any cause.
4. *Dystrophia myotonica.* A condition of unknown cause, in which a metabolic defect is presumed. It generally becomes apparent between 20 and 30 years of age and progresses slowly. Patients have a typically expressionless facial appearance with a slow, unrelaxing smile and bilateral ptosis. Other features include frontal baldness and genital atrophy. There is widespread neurological abnormality, characterized by inability to relax muscle groups, most strikingly found in the handgrip.

The patients become slow and apathetic. There is no known treatment for the underlying disorder, but visual impairment by cataract is usual by age 40, and the results of cataract surgery are good.

Syndromes of multiple congenital deformity

In Down's syndrome, characteristic cataracts appear about puberty.

Skin disorders

Cataract is associated with certain disorders of the skin — atopic dermatitis, for example.

Drugs

Steroids given over long periods, topically or systemically, may cause cataract — typically of the posterior subcapsular type which interferes markedly with vision.

Physical causes

1. *Trauma*. Injury to the lens capsule leads to opacification of lens fibres due to exposure to aqueous. A small hole in the capsule may lead to a limited opacity, but more severe injury leads to rapid opacification of the entire lens, which may swell, causing secondary glaucoma. Contusion, without rupture, can cause a characteristic rosette-like cataract, progressing rapidly to total opacity.

Treatment depends on the age of the patient, any associated injury and the state of the fellow eye. Surgery is usually indicated. Optical correction of the resulting aphakia may be provided, either by an implant or a contact lens, to restore binocular vision.

2. *Radiation*. Infrared, microwave and ionizing radiation and severe electric shock may cause cataract.

Secondary to other eye disease

Long-standing eye disorders such as chronic uveitis and persistent retinal detachment commonly lead to cataract.

Senile cataract

This is the most important group. Senile cataract is usually bilateral, though progression may be faster in one eye than the other. The exact biochemical cause of opacification of the lens is unknown.

Symptoms

The patient complains of failing vision. Apparently sudden deterioration may be due to a long-standing defect only recently noticed. The rate of progress is unpredictable. Cataracts of the nuclear sclerosis type, causing increase of refractive index in the nucleus of the lens, present with increasing myopia. Such patients, having required a presbyopic spectacle correction for reading, may enjoy a period in which they can read unaided.

Diagnosis

Visual acuity is reduced. Testing with a pinhole (p. 3) will eliminate refractive errors as the cause of the visual loss.

The diagnosis is made by examination of the eye with an ophthalmoscope through a dilated pupil. A cataract is most easily seen from a distance of about 30 cm with a +5 lens in the ophthalmoscope: the red reflex in the pupil is broken by opacities within the lens.

Treatment

Indications: Cataract surgery may be considered for any patient whose vision is significantly reduced in one or both eyes. There is no absolute level of acuity at which surgery should be advised or withheld. **Maturity** of a cataract is an absolute indication for its removal; a light directed obliquely at the pupil casts a shadow in the pupil unless the cataract is fully mature, when the entire pupil appears opaque. Complications, including lens-induced uveitis and glaucoma, are likely in the presence of an untreated mature cataract.

Surgical treatment

The enormous change in cataract surgery in the last two decades has been the development of intraocular lenses to substitute for the absence of the natural crystalline lens (aphakia). Intraocular lenses are now used in practically all cases except where there is a specific contraindication — for example, in chronic uveitis. Even high myopes benefit from the provision of a lens which accurately cor-

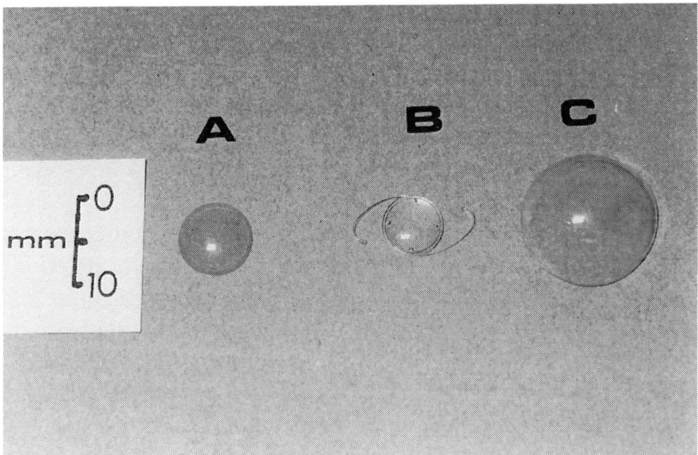

Fig. 8.2 Types of lenses: contact and intraocular

rects the eye to a satisfactory postoperative refractive state. The power of the lens implant required to give the desired postoperative refraction can be determined by biometry (p. 161).

Patients for whom lens implants are considered unsuitable must use alternative optical correction, by rigid or soft contact lens (Ch. 11) or 'aphakic' spectacles (Fig. 8.2).

Techniques of cataract surgery

A detailed discussion is inappropriate, but there are three regularly used methods of cataract removal.

1. *Extracapsular extraction.* Currently the most popular method, in which the anterior lens capsule is incised, the lens nucleus expressed, the cortex aspirated, and an implant inserted, usually into the 'capsular bag' (Fig. 8.3). The capsule remaining in front of the implant is then removed and the eye sutured with fine monofilament nylon. These sutures may be selectively removed in the follow-up period if they are causing distortion of the eye and astigmatism; otherwise, they dissolve 2 or 3 years later.

2. *Phakoemulsification.* Also known as 'one-stitch' cataract surgery, the technique is the same as in extracapsular extraction, except that the incision length is less than 4 mm and the lens nucleus is fragmented by a probe oscillating at ultrasonic frequency. Cortex aspiration follows. There must be a compromise in implant design if advantage is to be taken of the small initial incision, as the conventional implant is of 6 or 7 mm diameter.

The advantages of this method are quicker return to normal activity postoperatively, more reliable wound healing and less surgically induced astigmatism. Its disadvantages are in the need for more complex and expensive equipment, and the need to use an implant of less than the ideal diameter (or one that can be folded prior to insertion). The long-term results of the two methods are identical.

3. *Intracapsular extraction.* Formerly the most popular method, the trend is now away from the removal of the lens in its entirety because it is considered that a residual posterior lens capsule, apart from providing useful support for the fixation of the implant, confers protection from two potential complications of all cataract surgery — cystoid macular oedema, in which fluid collects at the macula in the first few weeks after operation, with impaired visual acuity, and aphakic retinal detachment.

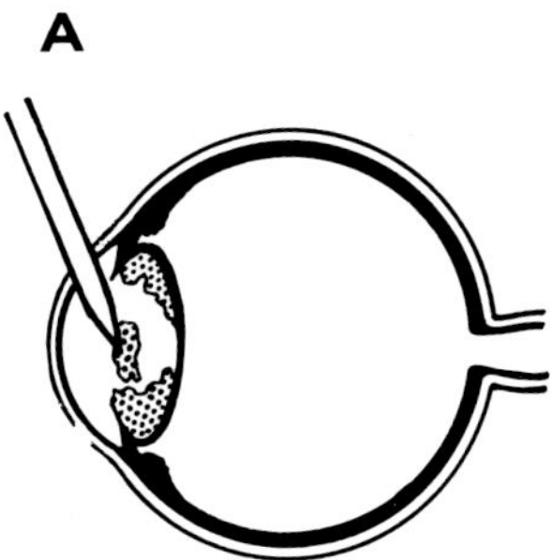

Fig. 8.3a Removal of lens matter from within capsule envelope

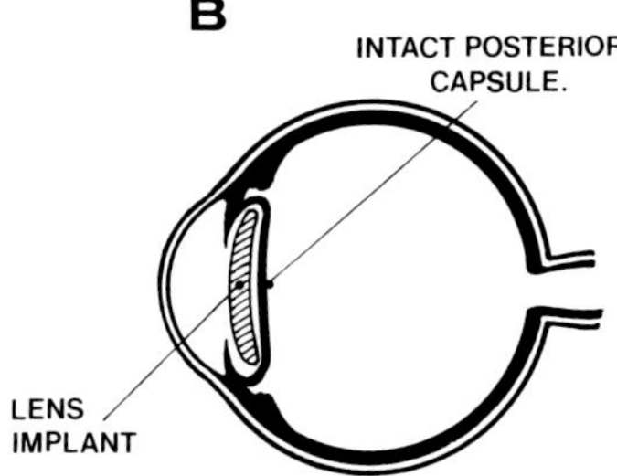

Fig. 8.3b Lens implant with anterior capsule removed and posterior capsule intact

If an implant is inserted following intracapsular extraction it is usually supported in the angle of the anterior chamber, so lying in front of the iris. The advantage of intracapsular surgery is that there is no residual posterior capsule to become opaque subsequently, with recurrence of visual impairment.

All three methods give excellent results and, with proper selection of cases, the outcome of modern cataract surgery can be virtually assured. Anaesthesia can either be local, with retro- or peribulbar injection of a long-acting agent, with or without basal sedation, or general. The operation can be undertaken as a 'day case' procedure, or by admitting the patient to hospital. No patient in whom there is an indication need be considered too old or frail for cataract removal.

Follow-up

The advice given to the patient after cataract surgery is a matter for the individual surgeon, but the general practitioner is likely, from time to time, to become involved.

The recovery period after surgery, whether undertaken as an in-patient or day case, is about 6 to 8 weeks, after which eyedrops are no longer required and definitive glasses are prescribed. Any patient with a painful or discharging eye, particularly with worsening vision, may have an intraocular infection and should be referred back to hospital forthwith. Such cases are, happily, rare. It is not unusual for the eye to be inflamed and mildly irritable postoperatively. Most surgeons prescribe steroid/antibiotic eyedrops for the first few weeks, and the general practitioner will be asked to renew this prescription as necessary.

Traditionally, postoperative cataract patients were advised not to stoop, have their hair washed, and so on; these restrictions are unnecessary with modern suturing techniques. Patients are now advised to avoid vigorous activity, such as digging the garden and moving heavy furniture, but the average elderly cataract patients need simply to be a little careful during the first few weeks. They may drive, providing they are comfortable and have adequate vision in the unoperated eye.

POSTERIOR CAPSULE OPACIFICATION

It is essential that the general practitioner understands that, following cataract surgery in which the posterior lens capsule is preserved (1 and 2 above), this may subsequently become opaque. This change may be regarded more as part of the healing process than as a complication of surgery, but its effect is to lead to gradual deterioration of vision in an eye which, after operation, had good sight. The incidence of capsular opacification is high in younger patients; less so after 70 years of age.

Treatment

Posterior capsular opacification is readily treated by YAG laser capsulotomy. This is an out-patient procedure and complications are rare. It is best postponed until at least 3 months after cataract surgery, if the protective benefits of the extracapsular technique are to be realized (see above) (Fig. 8.4).

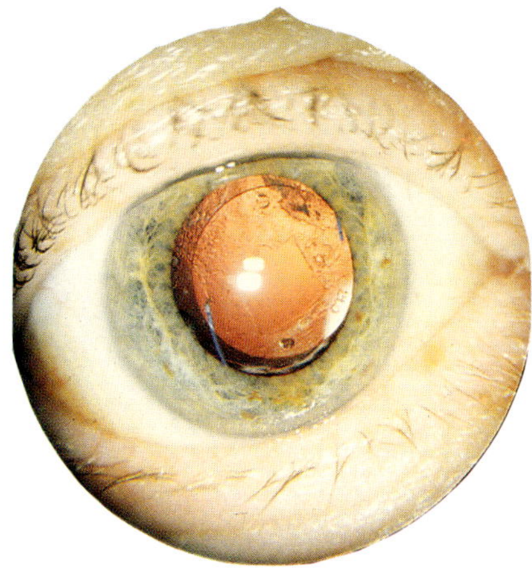

Fig. 8.4 Posterior capsule opacification (with laser capsulotomy)

The general practitioner must be vigilant and refer patients whose vision has deteriorated months or even years after successful cataract surgery. This applies particularly to the older and less articulate. They may otherwise become increasingly and unnecessarily blind in the belief that, having undergone surgery, nothing further can be done.

Once the posterior lens capsule has been opened by laser it will not become opaque again. The cause of any subsequent visual loss is likely to lie in the retina (Ch. 9).

SUTURE DISINTEGRATION

Nylon sutures, used to close the incision, may become loose or disintegrate at any time up to several years postoperatively. The patient complains of discomfort and may have a red eye. Referral to the hospital or surgeon quickly solves the problem.

9. The retina and vitreous

ANATOMY

The retina develops as an outgrowth of the forebrain and is invaginated to form two layers. The outer becomes the retinal pigment epithelium, and the inner the sensory retina, with the rods and cones adjacent to the pigment epithelium and the nerve fibre layer innermost.

At the posterior pole is an oval area some 5 mm in diameter — the macula. It contains a yellowish pigment. The central area of the macula, the fovea, contains cones, but no rods. The fovea lies about 3 mm temporal to the optic disc and has, at its centre, a depression, 0.4 mm in diameter, the foveola. Here the cones have no overlying layer except the internal limiting membrane. The healthy fovea gives a bright light reflex when seen with an ophthalmoscope. It is only at the macula that detailed visual discrimination, such as reading fine print, is possible.

The blood supply of the retina is from the central retinal artery, except at the fovea where the tissues are nourished from the innermost layer of the choroid — the choriocapillaris. The central retinal artery divides into four main branches, each accompanied by a tributary of the central retinal vein. The diameter of each vein exceeds that of the corresponding artery in a 3:2 ratio. Where they cross there is, in the normal fundus, no interference with the direction of either vessel.

The vitreous is a transparent gel with a collagenous fibrillary structure, occupying the posterior segment of the globe. In the healthy eye of a young person the vitreous is in contact with the entire retina, being attached at its periphery — the ora serrata — and at the optic disc. Passing across the vitreous from the disc to the posterior lens surface is the embryonic hyaloid vessel system. With ageing, particularly in myopic eyes, the vitreous undergoes liquefactive change — syneresis. In the elderly the periphery of the vitreous commonly becomes detached from the retina and optic disc, and the hyaloid remnants are visible to both patient and observer as a large 'floater'.

ARTERIOSCLEROTIC AND HYPERTENSIVE RETINOPATHY

Arteriosclerosis is seen in the retinal vessel walls (Fig. 9.1). The changes are most obvious at the arteriovenous crossings: the arterial walls lose their transparency and obscure the view of the underlying vein on either side of the column of blood. Further changes lead to pallor of the arterial light reflexes, more marked crossing changes, greater tortuosity of the larger vessels and a change of direction at the crossing from the normal oblique angle towards a right angle. The vein distal to the crossing may be dilated.

Advanced arteriosclerosis shows as marked pallor of the arterial light reflex and irregularity of the lumen, with yellowish staining of the vessel walls, like the stem of a clay pipe. The blood column disappears completely in places. In extreme cases the vessels may appear to be completely occluded, though their patency can be shown by angiography.

HYPERTENSION (Fig. 9.2)

Younger patients show narrowing of the arterioles. Prolonged hypertension leads to structural changes in the vessel walls, the hypertrophied smooth muscle being replaced by fibrous tissue. Older patients in whom there is significant arteriosclerosis show arteriovenous crossing changes and irregularity of arterial calibre. More severe hypertension may result in further retinal changes — haemorrhages, 'hard' exudates, retinal infarcts (cotton wool spots, or 'soft' exudates) and disc oedema.

Retinal haemorrhages in hypertension are most frequently seen in the superficial, nerve fibre layer of the retina. They may be linear or flame shaped and are most numerous near the optic disc. Haemorrhages confined to one sector of the fundus signify localized retinal vascular occlusion (see p. 87). Haemorrhages seldom interfere with vision unless one occurs at the macula.

'Hard' exudates are yellowish-white deposits in the deeper layers of the retina. They represent accumulated fat deposits and the residue of oedema. Their size varies from small dots to areas greater

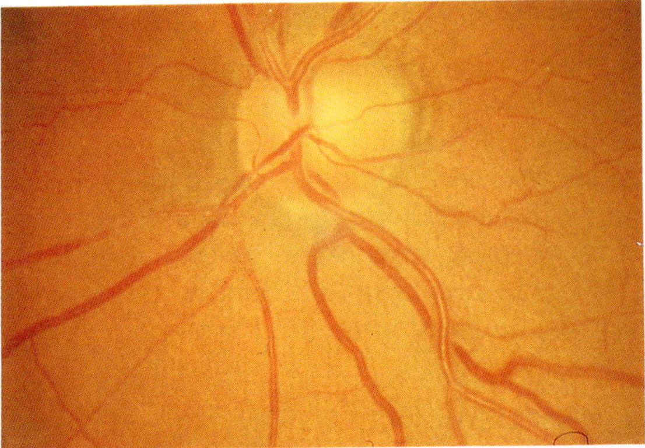

Fig. 9.1 Retinal arteriosclerosis

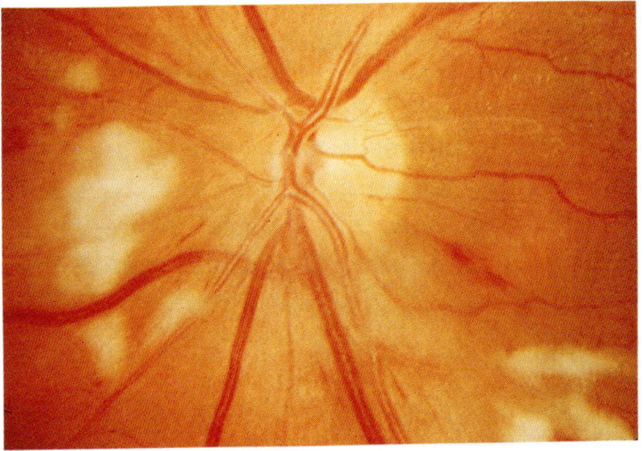

Fig. 9.2 Hypertensive retinopathy

than the diameter of the disc. They are commonly found in the region between the disc and the macula and in a star formation around the macula.

'Cotton wool' spots are retinal infarcts in the nerve fibre layer: they are accumulations of degenerate axoplasm. The term 'soft' exudate has largely been abandoned to avoid confusion with 'hard' exudates. 'Cotton wool' spots occur in the most severe forms of hypertensive retinopathy and indicate a grave prognosis. They are also seen in other systemic disorders — for example, diabetes (see p. 95), collagen disorders, blood dyscrasias and the acquired immune deficiency syndrome, AIDS (p. 101).

Optic disc oedema

Since the classification of hypertensive retinopathy by Keith, Wagener and Barker (1939), oedema of the optic disc has been regarded as the surest indication of severe hypertension. Optic disc oedema, cotton wool spots and flame-shaped haemorrhages indicate accelerated ('malignant') hypertension. The coexistence of other features of hypertensive retinopathy and the relatively slight elevation of the optic disc help differentiate this condition from papilloedema due to raised intracranial pressure.

RETINAL VASCULAR OCCLUSION

Central retinal artery occlusion

Failure of the retinal circulation leads to sudden and profound visual loss. If the occlusion persists, the ischaemic retina sustains irreversible damage, with swelling of the inner retinal layers due to accumulation of degenerate axoplasm. Usually occurring in the elderly, central retinal artery occlusion may be due to an embolus from the carotid or to thrombosis of an already arteriosclerotic vessel. The presenting symptom is sudden, painless loss of vision in one eye. Examination shows the absence of direct pupillary light reaction (see p. 7) and pale, attenuated retinal vessels. With progressive retinal damage, generalized retinal oedema is seen, ex-

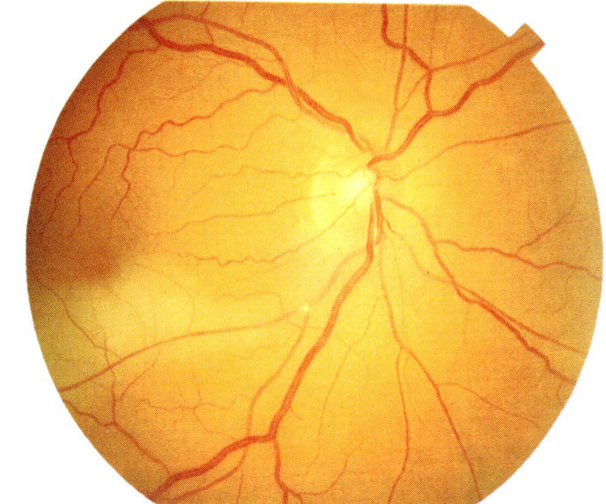

Fig. 9.3 Retinal branch artery occlusion: embolic occlusion of retinal arteriole. Note pale, oedematous retina distal to the embolus and contrasting 'cherry red' appearance around the fovea

Table 9.1 Investigation of central retina artery occlusion

General	Blood
Blood pressure	Full blood count ESR/blood viscosity
Urinalysis	Blood glucose Blood urea Syphilis serology Blood lipids
ECG Chest and skull X-rays Duplex carotid ultrasonography *or* i.v. digital subtraction angiography (Selective carotid angiography)	

Investigation of carotid blood flow — see also Chapter 16.

cept at the macula. Here the retina is thinnest and the area appears as a reddish spot owing to the visibility of the underlying choroidal circulation.

Unless the occlusion was caused by an embolus which passed into a more peripheral vessel, relieving the central obstruction, visual loss is permanent and optic atrophy becomes apparent after a few weeks. The retinal oedema subsides. There may be an audible carotid bruit.

Table 9.1 indicates the various tests required in the investigation of central retinal artery occlusion.

Management in the first few minutes consists of attempting to lower the intraocular pressure to encourage the onward passage of any embolus. Firm massage of the globe through the closed lids is the most effective treatment available to the general practitioner. The patient should be referred for ophthalmological assessment and review of the carotid arteries and cardiovascular system.

Retinal branch arterial occlusion

Also presenting as sudden, painless loss of vision, the portion of the visual field lost depends upon the extent of retinal arterial closure (Fig. 9.3).

Amaurosis fugax

Transient occlusion of the central retinal artery or one of its branches gives rise to 'fleeting blindness'. The patient usually complains of a 'curtain' obscuring vision for a few minutes. This is a form of transient ischaemic attack and is often the precursor of a major cerebrovascular accident. An embolus may be visible in one of the retinal arterioles. Giant cell arteritis (p. 146) is a less common cause: the diagnosis depends on finding a raised ESR and can be confirmed by temporal artery biopsy.

A carotid bruit should be sought by auscultation over the carotid bifurcation, at the level of the upper border of the larynx. Significant carotid stenosis may be present in the absence of a bruit and non-invasive techniques are available to study flow and turbulence: these include duplex carotid ultrasonography and intravenous digital subtraction angiography. Selective intra-arterial cerebral angiography is indicated in patients in whom carotid endarterectomy would be considered; it entails a risk of disabling stroke of about 1%.

Aspirin 300 mg daily is often recommended to reduce the likelihood of further transient ischaemic episodes. Attention must be paid to the control of all risk factors for stroke and myocardial infarction, including hypertension and smoking habits.

Central retinal vein occlusion

Occlusion of the vein has a less sudden presentation than that of the artery, owing to the variable element of ischaemia that accompanies venous obstruction. Visual loss is usually profound, developing over a period of hours or days.

The fundus appearance (Fig. 9.4) is typically dramatic, with extensive haemorrhages throughout, often as if red paint had been thrown at the retina; there may be numerous 'cotton wool' spots. Secondary glaucoma may occur about 3 months later (p. 144). Retinal new vessels may develop and subsequently give rise to vitreous haemorrhage.

Aetiology

Central retinal vein occlusion is predominantly a disease of the elderly. More than 60% have high blood pressure, and generalized cardiovascular disease and diabetes are also commonly found. Raised intraocular pressure, with or without established open-angle glaucoma, is also an important aetiological factor. Haematological

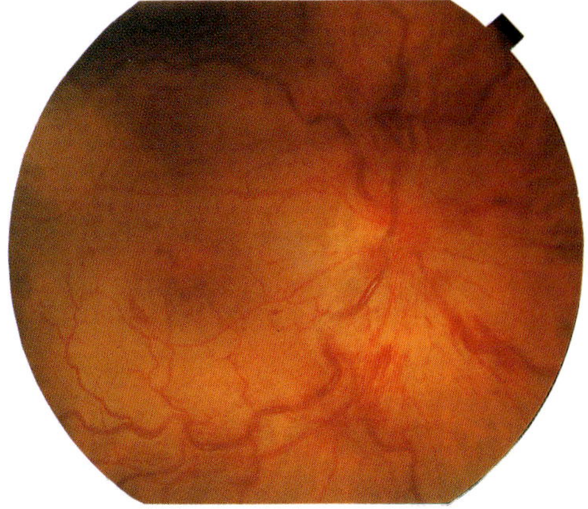

Fig. 9.4 Central retinal vein occlusion

factors such as dysproteinaemias and blood dyscrasias should be excluded. Oral contraceptives may be a contributory cause.

Every case should be referred for ophthalmological assessment as well as medical screening. The ophthalmologist may decide to investigate the retinal circulation by fluorescein angiography (see p. 160) to decide whether laser treatment is likely to prevent secondary thrombotic glaucoma. The most helpful factors in the patient's management are the correction of hypertension and other treatable circulatory and biochemical abnormalities.

Retinal branch vein occlusion

Occlusion of part of the retinal venous circulation occurs more commonly than central vein occlusion, and usually affects one of the vessels on the temporal side. Occlusion is distal to a crossing point, and haemorrhages and cotton wool spots are confined to the affected area of the fundus. If the macula is involved, central vision will be affected; otherwise the condition may pass unnoticed by the patient and be found at a routine fundus examination.

The aetiology is the same as that of central retinal vein occlusion and the patient should be similarly referred for investigation.

Vitreous haemorrhage

The symptoms of vitreous haemorrhage vary from the appearance of a few spots before the eye to sudden, complete, and painless visual loss. The diagnosis is made by finding blood in the vitreous on examination with a 'plus' lens in the ophthalmoscope — or by being able to see nothing at all with the instrument, if the haemorrhage is severe and the vitreous totally opaque.

Vitreous and other intraocular haemorrhages may occur spontaneously in perfectly healthy people, especially on severe exertion or the performance of a Valsalva manoeuvre. Trauma is also an important cause; but apparently spontaneous vitreous haemorrhage requires urgent referral in case there are other abnormalities within the eye.

Diabetes, hypertension and blood dyscrasias must be excluded and the patient investigated to identify treatable vascular disease. Full fundus examination should be carried out by an ophthalmologist at the earliest opportunity. If retinal details cannot be seen satisfactorily, the patient is kept under periodic review until, with clearance of the haemorrhage, a view of the fundus is obtained.

A number of retinal disorders may present with haemorrhage into the vitreous — a retinal tear or detachment, retinal vein occlusion or localized vascular abnormality. New vessel formation associated with vein occlusion, diabetes, sickle cell disease or retinal vasculitis may be found. Their diagnosis is a matter for the ophthalmologist.

Persistent vitreous haemorrhage may be treated surgically, by vitrectomy.

MACULAR DISORDERS

These may profoundly impair central vision but leave peripheral, navigating vision unaffected. The patient's symptoms will alert the general practitioner to the likely cause, but he may not have available sufficiently detailed examination techniques to make a confident diagnosis and most cases will therefore need to be referred. Pupillary dilatation with a short-acting mydriatic such as tropicamide 0.5% is essential for a satisfactory view of the macula.

An acute macular disturbance will usually impart 'kinks' to straight lines, and make objects seem smaller (micropsia) or larger (macropsia) than they appear with the other eye, owing to displacement of the foveal cones. The pupillary light reaction is unaffected, in contrast to disorders of the optic nerve in which there may also be profound loss of visual acuity with preservation of the peripheral visual field (see p. 147).

A complete list of macular disorders is inappropriate, but they may be classified according to likely age of onset.

Genetically determined macular disorders presenting in childhood

The commonest in this rare group of disorders is Stargardt's macular dystrophy. Children with initially normal visual development show progressive impairment of acuity to 'counting fingers' in the second decade and characteristic yellowish lesions appear at the posterior pole. Inheritance is recessive and both sexes are equally affected. Management consists of provision of low visual aids.

Macular disorders in early adult life

Central serous chorioretinopathy typically affects males and presents with impairment of vision in the third and fourth decades. Full recovery is usual, though many cases relapse — some repeatedly. The cause is leakage of fluid through a defect in the layer beneath the pigment epithelium, Bruch's membrane. The diagnosis may be confirmed by fluorescein angiography. Laser treatment is sometimes helpful in persistent cases.

Serous detachment of the retina localized at the macula may be associated with other ocular disorders such as a pit in the optic disc.

Myopic macular degeneration

High myopes are prone to various retinal disorders, including profound central visual impairment due to degenerative change at the macula. The choroid and retina become progressively atrophic and extensive areas of white sclera are exposed to view with the ophthalmoscope. It is usually difficult to examine the fundus of a highly myopic eye with a direct ophthalmoscope, but a better view may be obtained if the patient wears his glasses.

While macular degeneration is unlikely to be treatable, it is important to exclude retinal detachment involving the macula, and referral is therefore essential.

Age-related macular degenerations (Figs 9.5 and 9.6)

Age-related macular degeneration is the commonest reason for blind registration in developed countries.

Age-related *disciform macular degeneration* is a common form and is preceded by the appearance, at the macula, of yellow spots known as colloid bodies. Abnormal new vessels grow beneath the

Patient aged 71
Age-related macular degeneration

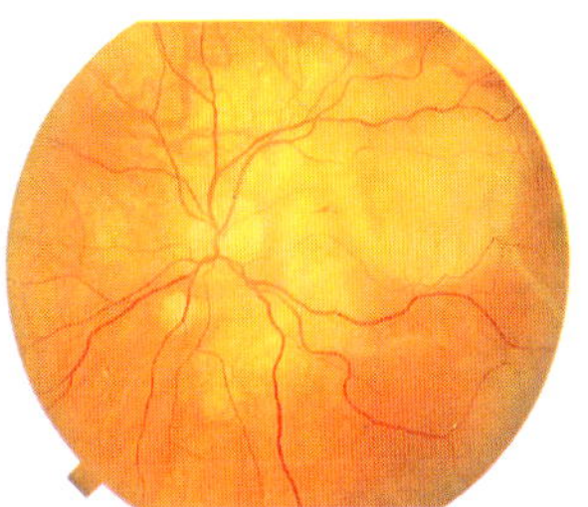

Fig. 9.5 Right eye
VA Hand movements

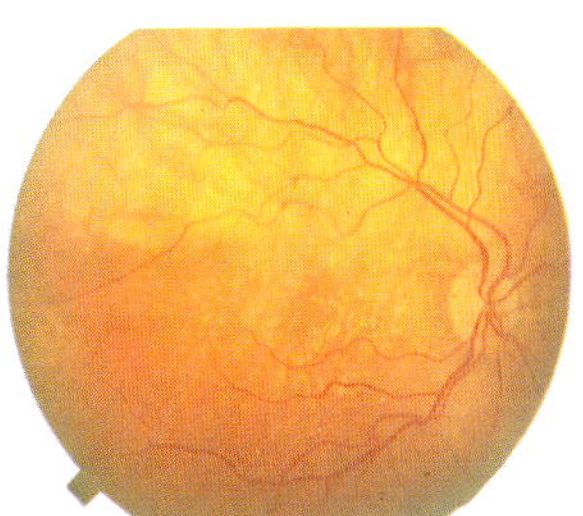

Fig. 9.6 Left eye
VA 6/9 (colloid bodies at macula)

retina from the choroid, and these leak, causing visual impairment made worse by subsequent scarring, so that the eventual acuity is reduced to 'hand movements'.

If the condition is recognized at an early stage and new vessels away from the fovea are identified by fluorescein angiography, the condition may be treatable by laser, preventing otherwise inevitable deterioration in vision. Successfully treated cases are uncommon, but the likelihood of the second eye becoming involved is about 20% per annum. It is therefore useful to warn the patient that symptoms arising in the second eye should be investigated early. Some ophthalmologists give patients already affected in one eye a test card known as an Amsler Chart, to check the central vision daily.

The whole disciform process evolves in a few weeks.

Retinal pigment epithelial detachment is a more benign form of macular degeneration which cannot be treated. A change of glasses may help, as the eye becomes relatively more hypermetropic. A scar or an atrophic area at the posterior pole of the eye is the likely outcome.

Age-related *macular hole* becomes bilateral in only about 10% of cases. Acuity is depressed to about 6/60.

Cystoid macular oedema may occur in diabetic retinopathy (p. 92) and after retinal vein occlusion (p. 87). Following cataract surgery it is frequently a transient event of little significance, though it may persist. Treatment is unsatisfactory and the visual outcome uncertain.

Patients with severe bilateral macular degeneration of any type usually maintain a fairly high level of independence. Appropriate advice and support are helpful and reassuring. For further discussion of blind and partially sighted registration, see page 167.

DRUG TOXICITY IN THE RETINA

Retinal damage may result from the prolonged administration of certain drugs — particularly chloroquine and some phenothiazines.

Quinine may cause rapid bilateral visual loss with dilated unreactive pupils. Recovery in a few days is usual.

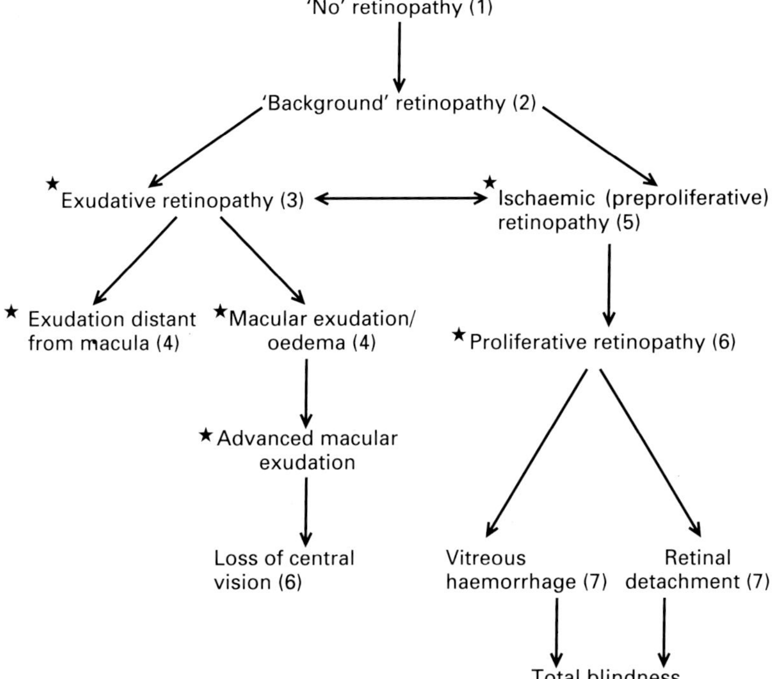

Fig. 9.7 Classification of diabetic retinopathy (the numbers refer to the listed text)

DIABETIC RETINOPATHY (Figs 9.8–9.11)

The exact cause of diabetic retinopathy is not known but experimental and clinical evidence shows that it is in part related to diabetic control. Never seen at the onset in young diabetics, retinopathy has an increasing incidence the longer the duration of diabetes. The elderly, maturity-onset diabetic may present with retinopathy or its complications before other symptoms of diabetes occur.

Classification

The object of any classification of diabetic retinopathy is to indicate:

1. The present state of the retinopathy
2. The need for treatment
3. The likely prognosis.

The underlying abnormality is in the walls of the small vessels in the retina, leading to local formation of microaneurysms, vessel leakage, exudation and capillary closure. Retinal ischaemia results in new vessel formation. Sight is damaged by oedema, exudation at the macula, haemorrhage arising from damaged and abnormal blood vessels, or by retinal detachment from fibrosis of new vessels and traction on the retina.

Management of diabetic retinopathy

Although prevention of retinopathy may be impossible, good control must always be the aim in managing diabetic patients. All diabetic patients, except juvenile-onset diabetics with disease of less than 5 years' duration, should have an annual examination after testing visual acuity and dilating the pupils of both eyes with a short-acting mydriatic (e.g. tropicamide 0.5%).

Laser or photocoagulation is now widely available and its introduction has fundamentally changed the management of diabetic retinopathy and made vigilant observation essential. Diabetics who are pregnant need to be watched with particular care.

Any doctor taking responsibility for the care of diabetic patients should ensure that the above requirement is fulfilled. If significant retinopathy is found the interval should be reduced to 6 months. Any case in whom retinopathy is other than 'background' or where either eye shows 'sight threatening' features should be referred for further assessment. Early treatment is far more effective than late. It is little use waiting for the patient to lose central vision in one

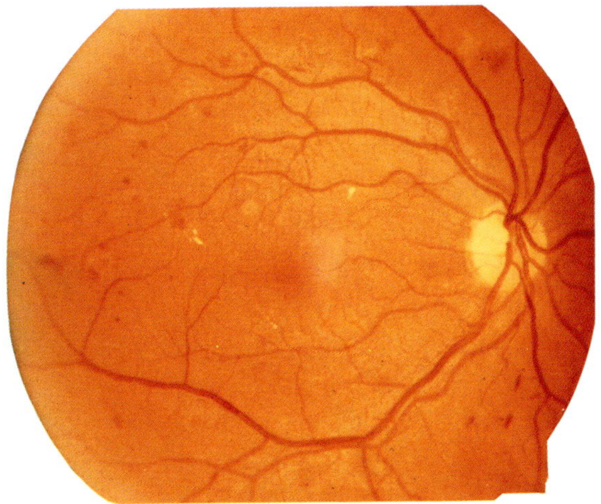

Fig. 9.8 'Background' diabetic retinopathy

eye before referring. Hypertensive and ischaemic changes may complicate diabetic retinopathy. Again, if in doubt, refer.

The categories shown in Figure 9.7 are considered below.

1. *'No' retinopathy*. The normal appearance of the fundi in diabetes is a safe indication that no retinal treatment is needed — at least until next year's follow-up. But fluorescein angiography of apparently normal eyes frequently shows extensive changes not visible on ophthalmoscopy — so there is little cause for complacency. Angiography is not necessary routinely.

2. *'Background' retinopathy* (Fig. 9.8). The earliest ophthalmoscopic changes in diabetic retinopathy are microaneurysms and haemorrhage. Microaneurysms appear as tiny red dots. The haemorrhages are characteristically of the 'dot' and 'blot' type which lie in the deeper layers of the retina. Hard exudates are also seen, though if they appear near the macula the classification of the fundus should be 'exudative' maculopathy and the patient referred. 'Background' retinopathy should be followed up every 6 months by the doctor managing the patient's diabetes.

3. *Exudative retinopathy/maculopathy* (Fig. 9.9). Significant 'hard' exudates constitute grounds for referral, particularly if they are near the macula. Typically, exudates accumulate in rings around a central area of microvascular leakage. Treatment of this area with

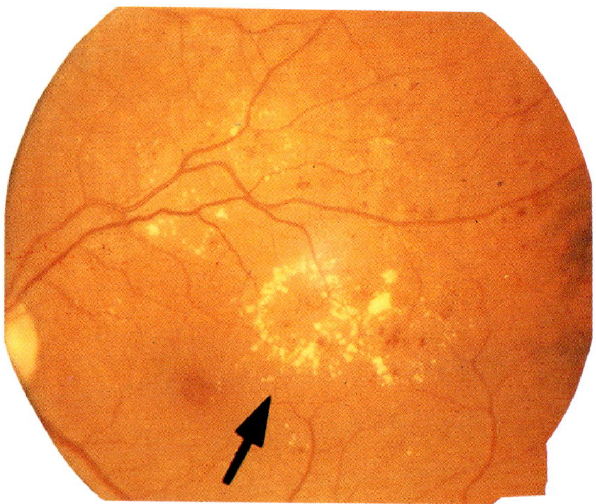

Fig. 9.9 'Exudative' diabetic retinopathy

laser coagulation usually causes the exudation to regress. Retinal tissue damaged by hard exudates does not recover its function, even though the exudation may disappear; hence the need for treatment before the onset of visual impairment. Macular oedema may be difficult to detect in the absence of hard exudates. Vision is impaired. Laser applications to the macula in a 'grid' pattern may reduce oedema.

4. *Advanced exudative retinopathy*. Irreversible damage to the macula results in permanent loss of central vision. The patient becomes eligible for blind registration if both eyes are affected, as in advanced senile macular degeneration, but useful 'navigating' vision is retained. Regular observation is still required in case the retina develops signs of proliferative retinopathy (see 5–7).

5. *Ischaemic (preproliferative) retinopathy* (Fig. 9.10). The signs of impending new vessel formation in the retina — and later the iris and anterior chamber (rubeosis iridis) with its disastrous consequences — are those of ischaemia of the tissues. 'Cotton wool' spots (retinal infarcts) are the cardinal sign, with distension of the veins into sausage-like segments and the formation of loops. Any suspicion of these changes or the appearance of new vessel networks either on the optic disc or peripherally demands urgent referral for laser treatment (see 6).

Treatment usually consists of the application of multiple laser burns (3000 or more) to the retinal periphery. The resulting overall reduction in the metabolic requirements of the retina removes the

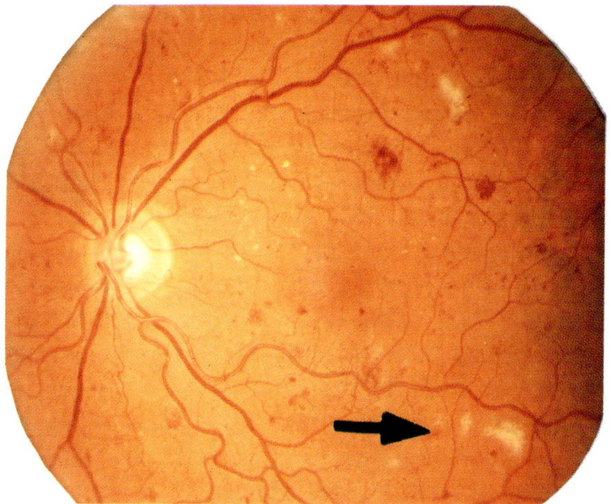

Fig. 9.10 'Ischaemic' diabetic retinopathy. Arrow indicates 'cotton wool' spots

stimulus to new vessel formation so that already developed new vessels regress and no more appear. The treatment is an out-patient procedure, often given in several sessions. Follow-up is likely to be carried out in the ophthalmic clinic after laser treatment.

6. *Proliferative retinopathy* (Fig. 9.11). New vessels, initially in the plane of the retina and subsequently growing forwards into the vitreous, are seen on the optic disc or elsewhere in the fundus.

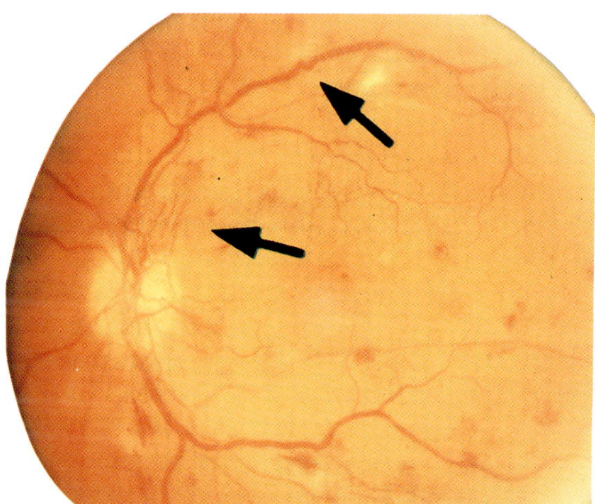

Fig. 9.11 'Proliferative' diabetic retinopathy. Arrows indicate new vessels and a venous loop

Their appearance indicates urgent need for referral and laser treatment. Failure to treat the retinopathy adequately at this stage leads inexorably to loss of vision (see 7).

7. *End-stage proliferative retinopathy*. Vitreous and subhyaloid haemorrhage and retinal detachment are disasters requiring referral. The usual practice with vitreous haemorrhage is to examine the eye by ultrasound 'B' scan (p. 162) to determine whether or not the retina is detached, and to wait for the haemorrhage to clear spontaneously. If it does not, and the ophthalmologist considers that the state of the underlying retina justifies surgery, the blood may be cleared by vitrectomy and the retina treated by photocoagulation from within the eye. Both this and the surgical treatment of diabetic traction retinal detachment by vitrectomy techniques are last-ditch procedures. Blindness resulting from proliferative retinopathy is, unlike the exudative type, usually complete.

Until more satisfactory metabolic management of diabetes prevents retinopathy — and the other vascular complications elsewhere in the body — regular, informed review of the fundi and referral for laser treatment as described above are the doctor's essential duty to his diabetic patients.

RETINOPATHY OF PREMATURITY (Retrolental fibroplasia)

Now rare in its fully developed state, retinopathy of prematurity reached epidemic proportions in the 1940s, before its cause was understood. In common with proliferative diabetic retinopathy, abnormal new vessels grow forward from the retina in response to ischaemia.

The administration of oxygen to premature babies with respiratory distress, resulting in high arterial Po_2, causes retinal vasoconstriction; if maintained, this becomes irreversible in 3–4 weeks. On reducing the oxygen concentration of the baby's environment, proliferative changes occur in the retinal circulation.

Infants thought to be at risk are usually examined by an ophthalmologist before discharge from the special care baby unit. The peak incidence of abnormalities is about 7 weeks after delivery. Most cases regress spontaneously, but more severe forms may be treated by cryotherapy. Since recognition of the cause, progression to retinal detachment and blindness is exceptionally rare.

RETINAL DETACHMENT (Fig. 9.12)

A common treatable cause of blindness, retinal detachment is of importance to the general practitioner because he may be consulted by patients with early symptoms when prompt referral and early treatment are all-important. He must therefore recognize the symptoms and signs.

The condition is misnamed. The detachment is that of the sensory retina (rods and cones) from the underlying pigment epithelium, with fluid accumulation between these parts of the retina — inaccurately termed 'subretinal' fluid. Detachment is usually associated with one or more breaks in the sensory retina.

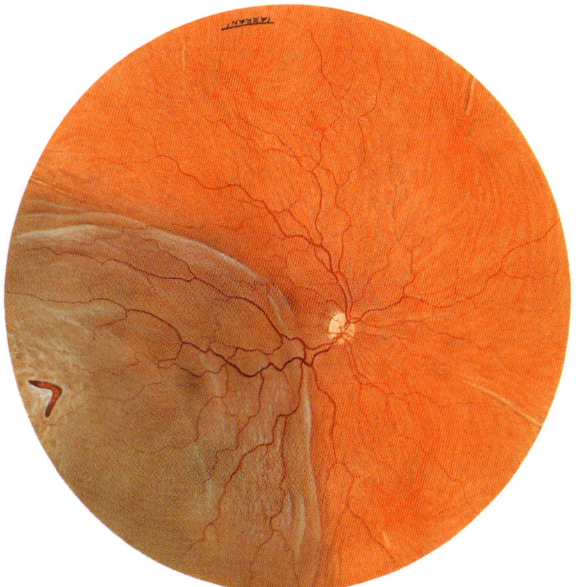

Fig. 9.12 Retinal detachment with retinal break

Diagnosis

Predisposing factors are myopia, particularly in the middle-aged, previous trauma, cataract surgery and a family history of retinal detachment.

Warning symptoms are 'flashing lights', associated with increased floaters, and spots before the eye. Retinal detachment causes a visual field defect corresponding to the area detached. The patient may complain of a 'curtain' across the vision. Any patient presenting with these symptoms should be sent for urgent examination by an eye surgeon even if no retinal detachment is seen. 'Spots' before the eye may signify a small vitreous haemorrhage if a retinal break passes across a blood vessel. When examined through a dilated pupil, the detached retina appears greyish-blue and may be ballooned forward into the vitreous, the vessels appearing blacker than those on the normal, attached retina.

The diagnostic problem in patients with symptoms suggestive of retinal detachment but no central visual loss is to distinguish 'innocent' degenerative vitreous changes from retinal breaks or early retinal detachment. At the ophthalmologist's disposal are more effective techniques for examining the peripheral retina — sometimes a very difficult task — and this responsibility should be passed on by the general practitioner.

Management

The retinal breaks are identified and are sealed by cryotherapy or other surgical means. Provided the macula is not involved at the start of treatment, excellent restoration of vision is usually possible. Established macular detachment inevitably leads to some impairment of function. Detachment of the superior retina, threatening to involve the macula, demands the most urgent surgical attention and the patient should lie flat until this can be achieved.

The patient should be able to return to work about 6 weeks after retinal detachment surgery, but contact sports and knocks on the head should be avoided indefinitely.

Retinal breaks without detachment may constitute a threat and the ophthalmologist must assess the risk and, where necessary, use laser or cryotherapy to the breaks or other signs of retinal degeneration. There is a significant risk of detachment in the second eye and this is always carefully examined and, if necessary, treated prophylactically.

RETINAL DETACHMENT WITHOUT A RETINAL BREAK

Intraocular tumours, particularly malignant melanoma, may produce retinal detachment below the tumour. The detachment is likely to be the presenting feature by causing loss of vision, the tumour itself having previously been unnoticed.

Exudative, serous detachment may also occur in systemic disorders such as renal failure and ocular inflammatory disorders such as scleritis.

RETINOSCHISIS

In contrast to retinal detachment, retinoschisis is a split developing between the layers of the sensory retina. The photoreceptors remain in contact with the underlying pigment epithelium. The condition is not uncommon, generally does not progress beyond the equator of the eye, and seldom requires treatment. Cases are found by opticians at routine refraction examination. It is advisable to seek specialist confirmation of the diagnosis.

ECLIPSE BURN OF THE MACULA

Rarely occurring now, ill-advised observation of an eclipse of the sun produces a macular burn sufficient to reduce central vision permanently. Careless handling of a laser may cause a similar disaster.

INHERITED DISORDERS OF THE RETINA

Retinitis pigmentosa (Fig. 9.13)

Retinitis pigmentosa is the commonest of a group of disorders, often with systemic associations, presenting with night blindness and progressive visual field loss.

Inheritance

Retinitis pigmentosa may be transmitted as an autosomal dominant, recessive or X-linked recessive. About 50% of cases arise with no previous family history; most are probably autosomal recessive.

Presentation

Night blindness is the first symptom, usually appearing in childhood. The more severe cases — typically with recessive inheritance — become aware of visual field loss in the second decade,

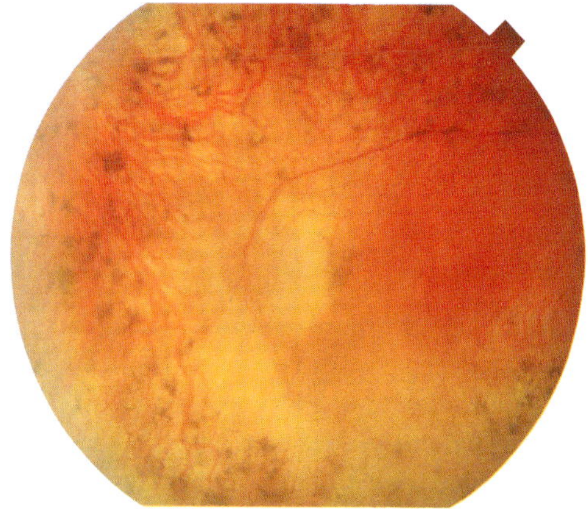

Fig. 9.13 Retinitis pigmentosa

and fundus changes are visible. Progressive field loss makes these patients blind by the fourth or fifth decade, although less severe forms of the disease may not interfere with vision until old age. Cataract may be a complicating factor.

Diagnosis

The fundus appearance is characteristic, with 'bone corpuscle' pigment clumping, particularly in the mid-periphery of the retina, attenuation of the retinal vessels and waxy pallor of the optic disc. Special testing of dark adaptation and of the electrical activity of the retina enable a diagnosis to be made in cases of doubt.

Management

No treatment is effective, but patients may be helped by suitable counselling, retraining and aids for the partially sighted or blind. Contact with the Retinitis Pigmentosa Society (p. 168) may be of comfort to many patients, and genetic counselling should be made available to those who request it. Patients with retinitis pigmentosa should not drive.

TUMOURS OF THE RETINA (Fig. 9.14)

Retinoblastoma is a rare and potentially lethal tumour, and may arise by spontaneous mutation or be inherited as an autosomal

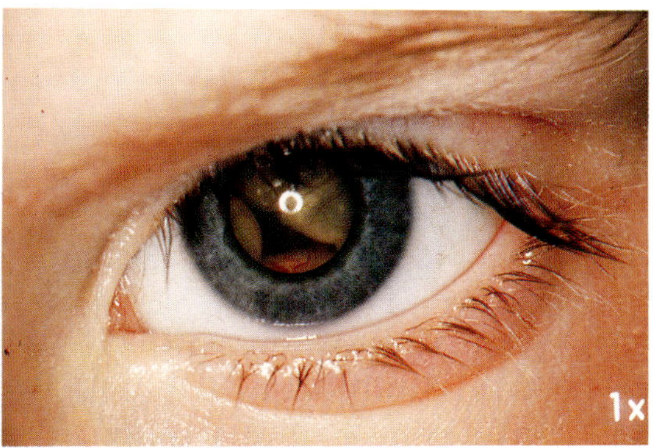

Fig. 9.14 Retinoblastoma

dominant. The diagnosis is usually made in the first 6 months of life by the appearance of a white mass in the pupil or a squint. Although conservative treatment may be possible, enucleation of the affected eye is usually necessary unless the diagnosis is made when the tumour is small.

Regular follow-up for the first 5 years is essential for the early detection and treatment of tumours arising in the fellow eye; about 30% are bilateral.

Any child with a persistent squint or a white mass in the pupil should be referred, the latter urgently.

INFLAMMATORY DISORDERS OF THE RETINA

Acquired immune deficiency syndrome (AIDS)

AIDS is a multisystem disorder caused by infection with the human immunodeficiency virus (HIV), and involvement of most parts of the body has been recorded. The ocular adnexa may be involved by Kaposi's sarcoma. The uveal tract, vitreous and retina may all be affected by opportunistic infections associated with 'full-blown' AIDS, and severe infections by both herpes simplex and herpes zoster, with their characteristic ophthalmic manifestations, are not infrequently seen.

The commonest sign of AIDS in the eye, and that most likely to be found by the general practitioner, is the appearance of a number of 'cotton wool' spots in the retinae of both eyes (Fig. 9.15). The mechanism by which these are produced is uncertain, but they

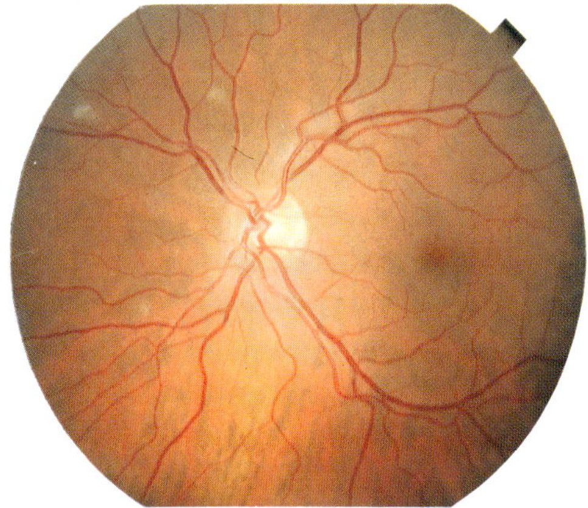

Fig. 9.15 AIDS (showing 'cotton wool' spots)

are thought to be a sign of intravascular clotting. 'Cotton wool' spots in the retina may appear in otherwise asymptomatic carriers of HIV infection.

Most dramatic are the haemorrhagic retinal lesions, described as 'cottage cheese and ketchup', due to retinal infection by cytomegalovirus. These may severely impair vision, but are unlikely to be encountered in general practice as they are a feature of the advanced stages of AIDS.

Other inflammatory disorders of the choroid and retina are considered on page 66.

10. Trauma

BLUNT INJURY

Without rupture of the globe

Such injuries are caused by fists, blows during sport, and a multitude of domestic and industrial mishaps. The effects range from a simple 'black eye' to gross disorganization of the globe.

The cornea may be abraded (see p. 51). Conjunctival lacerations merit referral because of the possibility of a concealed rupture of the globe.

Subconjunctival haemorrhage needs no treatment, provided vision is unimpaired.

Blood in the anterior chamber (hyphaema) shows as diffuse haziness of the aqueous, obscuring details of the iris and of the deeper parts of the eye. The blood settles to the lowest part where it lies with a characteristic fluid level (Fig. 10.1). Sometimes the anterior chamber becomes filled with blood. Admission to hospital is advised.

Traumatic mydriasis: persistent dilatation of the pupil due to damage to the iris sphincter is a not uncommon result of contusion. It generally recovers. Alternatively, the root of the iris may be torn (iridodialysis).

Traumatic cataract can follow contusion. In severe injuries, the lens is torn from its attachment, prolapsing forward through the pupil or falling back into the vitreous (subluxation or dislocation). The presence of gross visual defect will indicate major damage.

In the posterior segment, there may be bleeding into the vitreous or damage to the retina. Retinal oedema (commotio retinae) shows as a greyish area in the fundus where detail is obscured and there may be small retinal haemorrhages. It resolves with rest, though it is occasionally followed by pigmentary retinal changes and permanent visual loss. The retina may be torn by the distortion of the

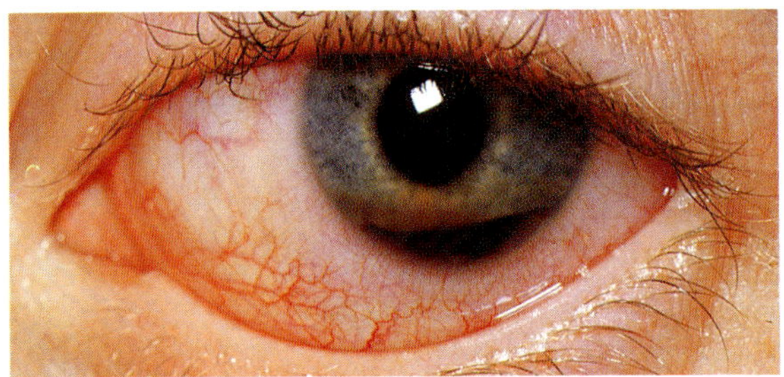

Fig. 10.1 Hyphaema

eye at the time of the injury, leading to retinal detachment. This may be delayed for months or years. Treatment is surgical (see p. 98).

Choroidal tears are sometimes seen and appear as scars, concentric with the disc and close to the posterior pole. These represent areas of choroidal atrophy through which the white sclera is visible.

Rupture of the globe

Sometimes the coats of the eye are not able to resist the pressure at the moment of impact, and rupture occurs, most commonly at the junction of cornea and sclera. There will be haemorrhage within the eye. Examination will show the rupture and there will usually be ocular contents presenting in the wound. Vision is grossly impaired and these injuries are unlikely to be missed unless lid swelling prevents adequate examination. Some attempt must always be made to examine the eye and to assess visual acuity. Defective vision, as in any eye problem, is the finding most likely to indicate the possibility of serious trouble.

PENETRATING INJURIES

Without retention of a foreign body

Potential causes include scissors, bows and arrows, darts, flying particles (particularly in industry) and windscreens. The resultant

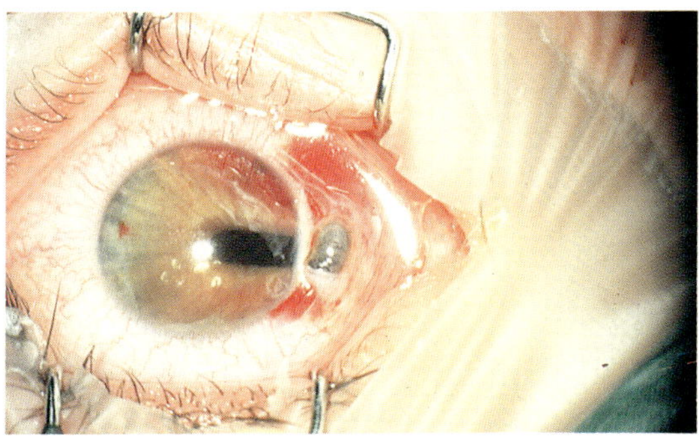

Fig. 10.2 Penetrating wound

injury is usually severe, though penetrations by such things as fine wire can be difficult to see.

There will be a history of something having struck the eye, which will be photophobic and watering and the vision impaired. If the wound is in the anterior part of the eye, the pupil is usually distorted and there may be prolapse of the iris through the wound (Fig. 10.2). Examination of the deeper eye is difficult on account of photophobia and haziness of the ocular structures. The lens may become opaque.

In a child, examination of the injured eye is particularly difficult. A child is sometimes loath to admit that he has sustained an injury. It may not be until the eye becomes red and painful during the subsequent days that the true position becomes apparent.

Treatment of these wounds is surgical, with wound toilet and repair. The prognosis for vision must be guarded.

With retention of a foreign body

These injuries are almost always industrial. Although provided with goggles, workers often fail to protect themselves adequately. The commonest cause is the hammer, striking a chisel or other metal tool. This throws off a steel flake which penetrates the eye. Travelling at high speed, these flakes are usually sterile and enter the eye through a small wound (Fig. 10.3). The worker may scarcely notice the incident, subsequently complaining simply that he got 'something in his eye'. This makes diagnosis difficult and those dealing with people engaged in work of this type should be constantly

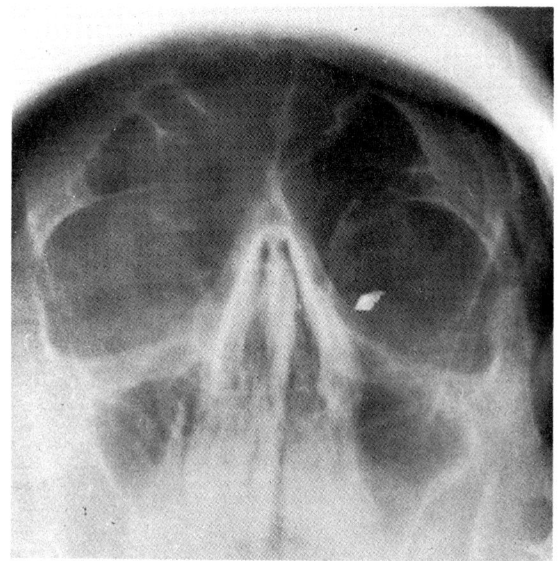

Fig. 10.3 Radiograph showing metallic intraocular foreign body

aware of the possibility of a penetrating injury if the foreign body is not visibly embedded in the surface of the cornea.

A piece of steel in the eye will, in the course of months or years, induce a chronic chemical reaction and will ultimately destroy sight (siderosis bulbi).

Examination may show a wound of entry, perhaps with prolapse of iris, and this is not likely to be mistaken. Difficulty arises if the entry wound is small, perhaps lying at the margin of the cornea, or in the sclera where it is covered by conjunctiva. A localized subconjunctival haemorrhage is a danger sign.

The cornea must be stained with fluorescein and the eye examined in a good light. Even if the entry wound is not visible, a hole in the substance of the iris is diagnostic of a foreign body retained within the eye.

The only sure diagnosis is by X-ray (Fig. 10.3), a routine in every case where the presence of an intraocular foreign body is suspected.

Treatment involves repair of the wound and removal of the foreign body after X-ray localization. Removal may be by magnet if the particle is of steel, or by vitrectomy.

Sympathetic ophthalmitis

This rare condition may follow a penetrating injury of the eye. Persistent inflammation in the injured eye leads to low-grade iridocyclitis in the fellow eye after 2 or 3 weeks or longer. This can be very destructive and difficult to control. The cause of the condition is poorly understood, but it represents a sensitivity reaction in the second eye. The decision as to whether or not an injured eye should be removed, in the face of a possible risk to the other eye, can be difficult.

INJURIES TO THE ORBIT

Orbital haematoma may follow contusion, and fracture of the orbital bones may displace or damage the extraocular muscles.

Double vision suggests the possibility of a 'blow-out' fracture (Fig. 10.4) and all contusion injuries leading to double vision should be referred. In 'blow-out' fracture an extraocular muscle becomes trapped in a fracture of the floor or, occasionally, the medial wall of the orbit. There is enophthalmos, due to prolapse of the orbital contents, and limitation of movement, usually on upward gaze.

The X-ray finding of a 'tear-drop' opacity in the antrum (Fig. 10.5) is characteristic of a 'blow-out' fracture of the orbital

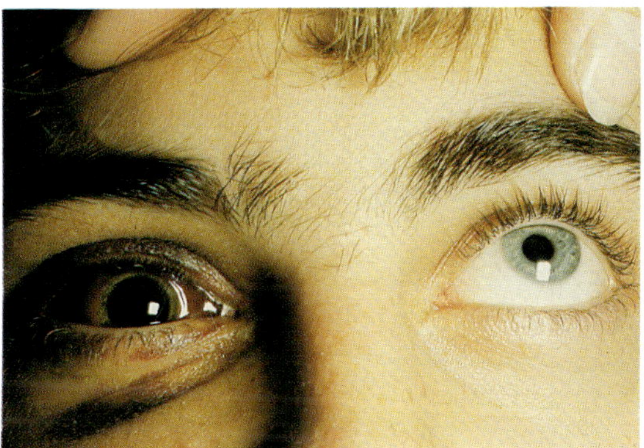

Fig. 10.4 'Blow-out' fracture

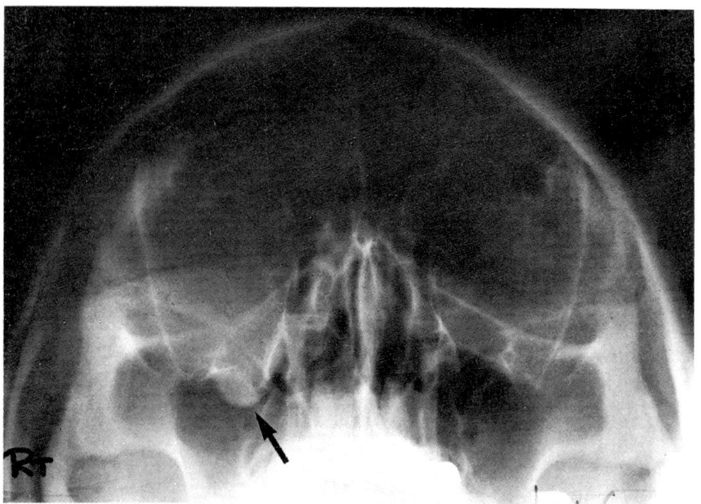

Fig. 10.5 Radiograph of blow-out fracture of orbit: note 'tear-drop' opacity in antrum

floor. The orbit may have to be explored to free the trapped muscle and cover the bony defect.

Occasionally a blow to the head may interfere with the delicate blood supply of the optic nerve as it passes through the optic canal, causing severe visual impairment in the affected eye. Optic nerve damage is indicated by an afferent pupillary defect (p. 7). Optic atrophy appears after a few weeks. There is no effective treatment. A squint, usually divergent, may develop later.

11. Spectacles and contact lenses

The formation of a clearly focused retinal image depends on the presence of a normal relationship between the axial length of the eye and the focal length of the lens system. The term 'lens system' is used because there are two elements involved in the refraction of light entering the eye. One is the biconvex lens and the other, more powerful from the optical point of view, the convex anterior surface of the cornea.

Accommodation

If the eye is to be given a clear image of objects at varying distances, it must adapt the focal length of the lens system to suit the varying angle of the entering rays. This is achieved by changing the curvature of the lens of the eye — accommodation.

Consisting of a transparent mass of lens matter enclosed in an elastic membrane, the lens capsule, the lens is supported within the circle of the ciliary body by a series of fine fibres, the zonule, or suspensory ligament.

The ciliary body contains a mass of muscle fibres innervated by the parasympathetic element of the third cranial nerve, and is able, by its contraction, to alter the tension in the suspensory ligament and thus in the lens capsule. Contraction of the ciliary muscle increases the curvature of the lens and so shortens its focal length.

The stimulus for accommodation is reflex, based on the need to maintain a clear retinal image (Fig. 11.1). There is a natural relationship between the accommodative effort required to produce a clear retinal image and the amount of convergence of the visual axes to keep the images on the maculae of both eyes. The importance of the balance between these two functions is considered in the discussion of errors of refraction in relation to the aetiology of squint (AC/A ratio).

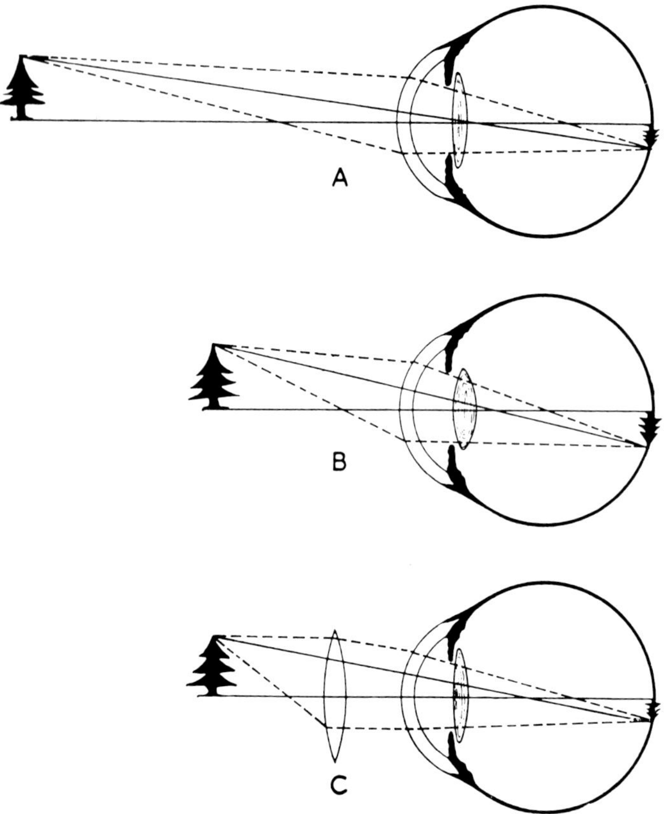

Fig. 11.1 Formation of the retinal image. (A) In the normal eye, with the accommodation relaxed, the image of a distant object falls on the retina. (B) When the object approaches the eye a change of shape of the lens takes place and the image remains focused on the retina. This is accommodation. (C) With increasing age the eye loses its power to change its focus for close objects and has to be reinforced by convex lenses to keep the image in focus. This is presbyopia.

Presbyopia

As age increases, the lens of the eye becomes larger and less able to respond to the efforts of the ciliary body to alter its curvature. At the age of about 45 reading and sewing become more difficult and by 65 all power of accommodation is lost.

The middle-aged must simply accept the need to wear glasses for close work. Whether these be bifocal, varifocal or simple reading glasses is purely a matter of choice.

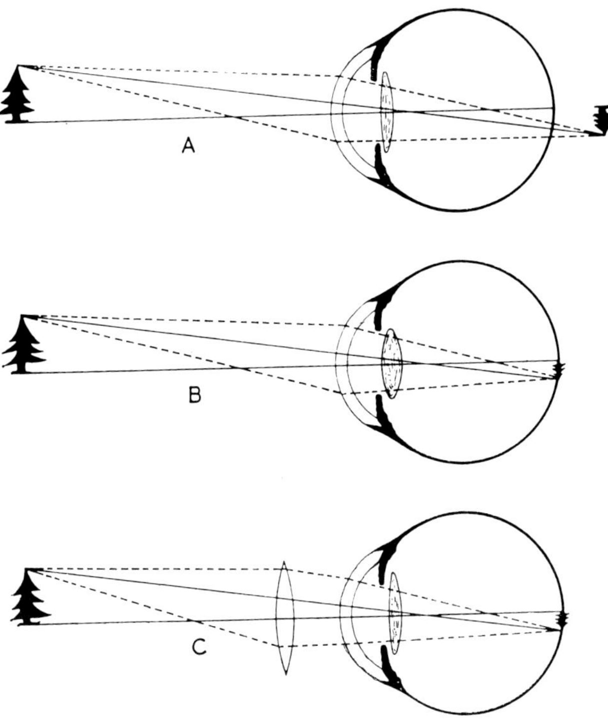

Fig. 11.2 Hypermetropia. (A) With the accommodation relaxed, the image of a distant object falls behind the retina. (B) An effort of accommodation is required for the clear viewing of an object, even in the distance. (C) This effort has to be increased as the object becomes closer. If the error cannot comfortably be overcome by accommodation, a convex spectacle will be needed.

Hypermetropia (hyperopia, long sight)

This is the commonest refractive error. Almost universal in infants, it becomes less in the growing years.

In hypermetropia, the accommodation being relaxed, rays of light from an object in the distance are brought to a focus behind the retina (Fig. 11.2). In youth, if the degree of hypermetropia is slight, this defect is no disadvantage as it can be overcome by accommodation — but reading may be an effort (see p. 110).

Hypermetropia needs correction only if it is of such a degree as not to be comfortably overcome by the use of the eye's own focusing mechanism. Exceptions are children with convergent squint or with amblyopia of one eye due to unequal refractive errors (p. 124).

A degree of hypermetropia insufficient to cause symptoms in

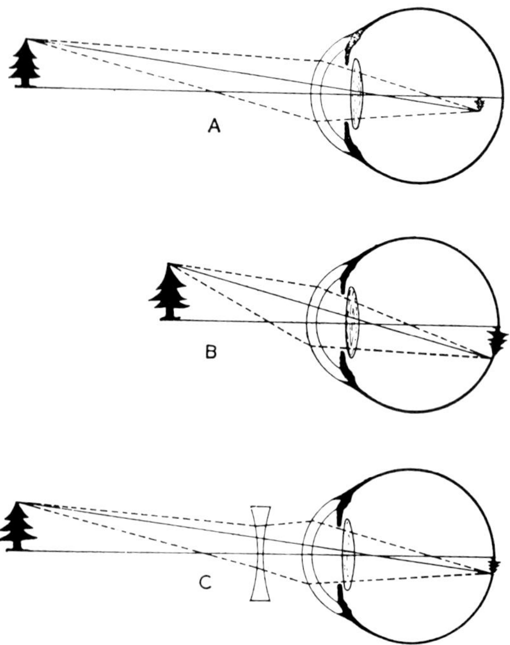

Fig. 11.3 Myopia. (A) The image of a distant object falls in front of the retina and any effort of accommodation will only increase the blurring. (B) Near objects, on the other hand, are seen clearly with little or no accommodation. (C) For clear distant sight, concave glasses are needed.

youth may, with the natural lessening of the power of accommodation, give rise to reading difficulties in middle life. There will be an earlier demand for reading glasses than in the patient with no refractive error — emmetropia.

Myopia (short sight)

In myopia, rays of light from a distant object are focused in front of the retina, either because the eye is excessively long or the refractive elements — cornea and lens — of too great a power to produce a clearly focused image on distance fixation (Fig. 11.3). The myope is at a disadvantage compared to the hypermetrope in that he is unable to obtain clear distant vision by the exercise of his accommodation. At close range, however, the advantage is with the myope, who can focus on near objects with little or no effort of accommodation.

Myopia is of two types: simple myopia, which is common, and progressive, or degenerative myopia, which is uncommon.

Simple myopia

Simple myopia is often hereditary. With growth, the globe becomes too long. The onset is usually about puberty, hence the term 'school short sight', but it may be delayed into early adult life.

The system of routine examination of schoolchildren generally leads to prompt recognition of the condition, or the teacher notices that the child is not reading the blackboard from the back of the class. In preschool children, parents complain that a child holds books very close to his face or sits too near the television.

Simple myopia advances during the school years and the need for new glasses can only be determined by regular examination. The child can then lead a normal life and can play most games — in splinterproof glasses or contact lenses. It is not essential that he wear his glasses from morning to night, as he probably will not take kindly to the idea of glasses in any case, but they should be worn in class and at other times when clear distant vision is required. As he grows older, he will decide for himself when glasses are to be worn.

Particular attention should be paid to the vision of siblings when there is a short-sighted child in the family. Measures to arrest or prevent myopia, apart from radial keratotomy (p. 119), have failed to gain general acceptance.

Degenerative myopia

A condition of unknown cause associated with very high degrees of myopia and with pathological changes within the eye. Among these are vitreous opacities, cataract formation and degenerative changes at the posterior pole of the eye, often leading to the destruction of central vision (p. 89).

Retinal detachment is more common in myopes than in normally sighted individuals, the incidence increasing with the degree of myopia.

Astigmatism

Astigmatism means that the curvature of the cornea is not the same in all meridia. It may be associated with either hypermetropia or myopia, and requires a cylindrical lens for its correction. Failure to correct higher degrees of astigmatism in the years of visual development may lead to partial amblyopia.

There are some pathological conditions which, by causing distortion of the cornea, produce irregular astigmatism. Among these are diseases of the cornea such as keratoconus, corneal ulceration of various types, tarsal cysts, and the results of injury.

Ocular headache

Headache is a very common complaint, and it is certainly prominent among the reasons for which patients are referred for an ophthalmic opinion. There are some features of headache which may point to the eyes being involved in a given case.

The ocular headache is often related to, or precipitated by, the use of the eyes. Thus it occurs on prolonged reading or sewing, watching television, or taking up a clerical occupation for the first time. The pain may be delayed in onset, appearing in the morning after an evening of ocular activity. It may be felt in the eyes themselves, or in the temple or occiput, in which case it is probably coming from the neck muscles.

Ocular headache is usually regular in occurrence. A pain appearing at long intervals, without any change of ocular habit, is not likely to be of ocular origin. The same can be said of a pain of recent onset, without there having been any change in the use of the eyes.

Sufferers from migraine often present with ocular symptoms — flickering lights, hemianopia, and so on — but the headache which follows is unlikely to be influenced by the provision of glasses.

Refractive changes in diabetes

About a third of diabetics, particularly those with higher levels of blood glucose, show a temporary change towards myopia at the onset of the illness. This can precede other symptoms by several weeks or months. Patients in the presbyopic age group may find their reading glasses unnecessary but their distance vision blurred. An unexpected myopic shift in refraction should suggest the possibility of diabetes and the urine should be tested for glucose.

Transient hypermetropia frequently occurs as the blood sugar level falls on starting treatment; glasses should not be prescribed until the condition has been stable for several weeks.

Contact lenses

Contact lenses may be used as an alternative to spectacles for the correction of all refractive errors. In general, the higher the refractive error, the greater the benefit of contact lenses, but their use on cosmetic grounds and on account of the unobstructed vision they provide constitute important reasons for many patients' preference for contact lenses instead of spectacles. Occasionally contact lenses are ordered as part of the treatment of eye disorders rather than on purely optical grounds; for example, in keratoconus where the astigmatism is too great to be corrected by spectacles, and in some cases of corneal ulceration, for protective purposes.

Contact lenses are of two main types, according to the material from which they are made: rigid and soft (hydrophilic).

Rigid lenses

Rigid ('hard') lenses are made of a variety of materials. Perspex, the standard for many years, has been overtaken in popularity by newer substances having less tendency to deprive the cornea of oxygen. Hypoxia leads to fluid retention within the corneal stroma and oedema of the epithelium which leads to discomfort and blurred vision.

Rigid lenses have to be fitted so as to minimize oxygen deprivation and, in general, their wear must be restricted so that the oxygen supply of the cornea can be replenished.

Problems. The commonest problems presented to the doctor by wearers of rigid contact lenses are associated with oxygen deprivation, usually caused by wearing the lenses too long, and minor trauma caused by their insertion or removal. Patients with problems associated with contact lens wear should be advised not to use the lens for 48 h. The wearing time should then be extended gradually, as most patients are advised when beginning to use lenses.

Infection is also a potential danger, though less than with soft lenses. The spectrum of damage extends from small, sterile corneal infiltrates consisting of aggregations of leucocytes, to severe, suppurative infection. Hygiene, with cleaning of both the lenses and their container, is important.

An apparently lost contact lens may sometimes be found in the superior conjunctival fornix on everting the upper lid (see p. 35).

Women taking oral contraceptives may have slightly impaired tolerance of contact lens wear.

Soft lenses

Soft, or hydrophilic, lenses conform to the curvature of the cornea and are classified according to the material of which they are made and to their water content, which may range from 40 to 90%. The materials of higher water content tend to permit greater diffusion of oxygen through the lens to the cornea. The lenses must always be kept in an appropriate storage solution. If allowed to dry they become distorted and brittle, and cannot be used until fully rehydrated.

Soft lenses are more widely used than the rigid type, and they have the advantages of longer initial wearing times and greater initial comfort. They produce less distortion of the cornea in use so they may be more readily interchanged with spectacles, allowing intermittent use — as, for example, in sport. Soft lenses are larger than the rigid type, usually overlapping the cornea by 1 to 2 mm. Certain soft lens materials allow extended wear for days, weeks, or even months. Those intended only for daily wear should be removed before sleep.

Problems. Sterility is of great importance with soft contact lenses as the material from which they are made can become contaminated by bacteria or by the protozoon *Acanthamoeba* (see p. 58). Care has to be taken when handling the lenses and the user should wash his hands before inserting or removing a lens. The lens is generally rubbed with a surface cleaning agent after removal from the eye and disinfected with chemicals or by heat. Soft lenses attract protein deposits and these are usually removed weekly by enzyme tablets.

Extended wear lenses carry the greatest risk of infection. Any infection is potentially serious and may lead to corneal ulceration and irreversible vascularization. Should infection be suspected, lens wear must be discontinued and appropriate antibiotic treatment instituted. The cornea must be checked by slit lamp examination before lens wear is resumed.

It is with disinfecting agents containing thiomersal that problems with soft contact lenses are most frequently associated. These agents are toxic in high concentrations and accumulate in the con-

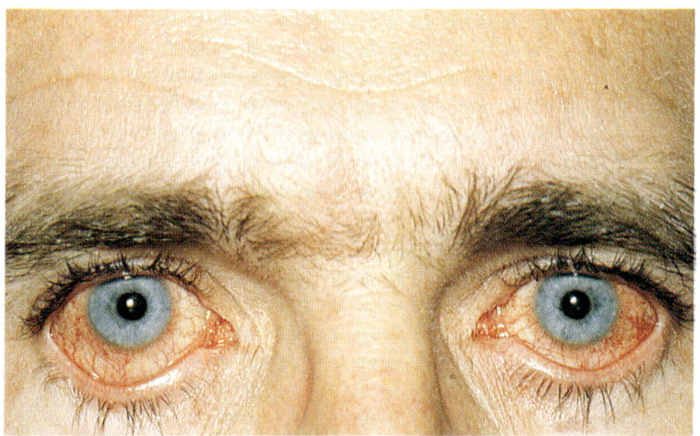

Fig. 11.4 Conjuctivitis due to contact lens solution.

tact lens. The symptoms of toxic effects of lens disinfectants are lens intolerance and discomfort. The signs are red eye, with hyperaemia and follicle formation, and hypertrophy of conjunctival papillae. A soft lens wearer who becomes intolerant of disinfecting chemicals is usually advised to change to boiling the lenses in normal saline without preservative, or to clean the lenses in hydrogen peroxide (Fig. 11.4).

Infection, with corneal ulceration, is a less common but serious problem. Ulceration can lead to corneal vascularization. Should this occur, soft lens wear must be discontinued until the ulcer has healed and all new vessels have regressed. Antibiotic drops are prescribed. Gradually increasing vascularization from the corneal periphery may also occur without infection — probably in response to hypoxia. Hence soft lens wearers should have a periodic slit lamp examination.

Soft lenses give less satisfactory visual acuity than rigid hard lenses if used to correct refractive errors which include significant degrees of astigmatism. They are also less durable and have to be discarded if damaged, discoloured or affected by protein deposition. Disposable soft lenses are now available which are used for a week or so and then discarded. Chemical agents are therefore unnecessary.

Technique for removal of a contact lens (Fig. 11.5)

A general practitioner may occasionally be called upon to remove a contact lens from an eye which, for any reason, is irritable or

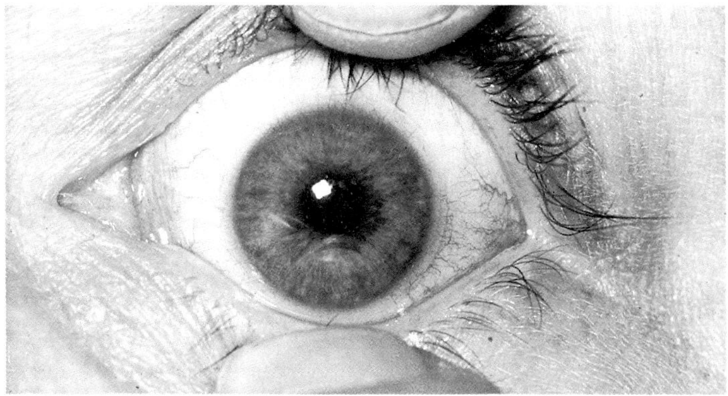

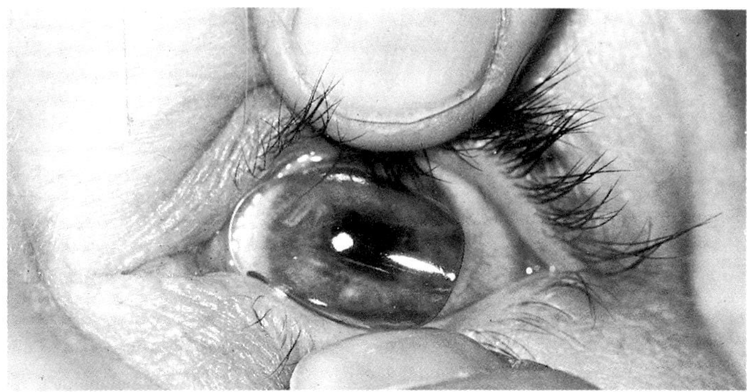

Fig. 11.5 Removal of a soft contact lens.

inflamed. For example, the elderly aphakic patient who has been fitted with an extended wear soft lens and who is unable to get to the specialist:

1. Open the eye widely with the index fingers behind the lashes of each lid.
2. Gently press the lid margins together so that they touch the edges of the contact lens. This will release the lens from the surface of the eye. It can then be picked off the lid margin.
3. If the first attempt is not successful, try again.

Tear production

Inadequate tear secretion is often a cause of poor tolerance of contact lenses of any type. This can be assessed by Schirmer's test (p. 31).

Drugs and contact lenses

Printed on the packets of some eyedrop preparations are the words: 'not to be used with contact lenses'. This is a controversial matter, and it applies to soft lenses. There are two possible reasons for advising against the use of certain eyedrops with contact lenses:

1. Because the drops may, in the long term, damage or discolour the contact lens.
2. Because the drops contain a preservative — commonly benzalkonium chloride — to which the lens wearer may develop an adverse local reaction.

However, lens preservative intolerance develops in only a few cases, and usually after at least 6 months' use. So on neither count need this advice be taken too seriously if the eye drops must be used and the patient insists on wearing the lens.

It is of greater concern that a contact lens is not worn when there is an eye disorder, such as keratitis or conjunctivitis, in which the lens might be implicated. 'When in doubt, take it out' is sound advice for any contact lens wearer.

REFRACTIVE SURGERY

Patients may seek the general practitioner's advice on this subject.

Corneal procedures

Permanent alteration of the refractive state of the eye by safe and predictable surgery has proved an elusive goal for ophthalmologists. The most frequently practised technique of refractive surgery is the selective removal or adjustment of corneal sutures where there is wound distortion after cataract surgery. This is generally done during the follow-up period — ideally within 2 months of the operation. Biometry permits the selection of a lens implant tailored to the desired postoperative refraction state (see p. 161).

Radial keratotomy is a procedure for the correction of myopia. Indications include intolerance of contact lenses, combined with a dislike of, or fear of losing, glasses, and a desire to improve the unaided visual acuity for occupational reasons or to make possible participation in outdoor sports such as skiing and mountaineering without optical aids.

The technique is to make, under topical anaesthesia, a number of radial incisions in the cornea to 90–95% of its thickness, avoiding the central, optical zone.

The results with lower refractive errors are excellent. Patients with up to 3 dioptres of preoperative myopia achieve an unaided visual acuity of 6/12 or better in 99% of cases, falling to 40% in the group with myopia of more than 6 dioptres.

Disadvantages include a period of unstable postoperative refraction due to increased flexibility of the cornea, which improves with time, and a small risk of overcorrection leading to hypermetropia. This becomes more significant with the onset of presbyopia over the age of 45. The myopic patient considering the operation must be aware of the relative advantage he will have foregone in his presbyopic years. Astigmatism may, rarely, be introduced by the procedure.

'Glare' caused by the central ends of the radial incisions occasionally causes a problem and there is the theoretical possibility that the cornea, weakened by surgery, may be more readily ruptured by direct trauma. Severe infective keratitis has very rarely been reported.

Prospective radial keratotomy patients with myopia in excess of 6 dioptres should not expect their refractive error to be eliminated, though it will be reduced. The greater risk of retinal detachment in myopes, due to the greater than normal axial length of the globe, is unaffected by the operation.

Medical officers in the United Kingdom Armed Forces have recommended that potential recruits who have had the operation of radial keratotomy should not be accepted for enlistment.

Epikeratophakia is another accepted technique of refractive surgery. Correction of high hypermetropic errors — particularly aphakia in subjects unsuitable for lens implantation — is achieved by suturing to the corneal surface a prepared disc of donor cornea. The operation is particularly useful in infants, in whom intraocular lenses are generally not used, and in aphakic patients with chronic uveitis who cannot have a lens implant and who may be unable to tolerate a contact lens.

Several other techniques are either in the development stage, or are very little used on account of their complexity. Sculpting of the corneal surface by *excimer laser* is one such procedure now emerging from the experimental stage, and results to date are promising.

Intraocular surgical procedures

Anterior chamber lens implants of negative power. For patients whose myopia is too great to be satisfactorily reduced by radial keratotomy, and who are intolerant of spectacles and contact lenses, an implant can be inserted without lens extraction. The early visual results are excellent but longer term complications remain uncertain, particularly with regard to the possibility of progressive corneal changes leading to decompensation and oedema — perhaps years later.

Clear-lens extraction is another procedure which has been tried; the principal disadvantage is an increased incidence of retinal detachment.

Neither of these approaches has yet achieved widespread acceptance.

12. Ocular motility

SQUINT (Strabismus)

A squint is present when the image of an object falls on the fovea of one eye but not of the other.

CLASSIFICATION

1. Non-paralytic or concomitant. The angle of deviation does not vary with direction of gaze.
2. Paralytic. The angle of deviation varies with direction of gaze.

Non-paralytic squint

The development of binocular vision

The central part of the retina, the macula, is the only part with which detail can be seen, and an inborn reflex normally brings the image of an object on to the fovea.

The eyes are aligned in order to avoid double vision. If an obstacle makes the binocular use of the eyes difficult, the child disregards the image seen by one eye and concentrates on the other. Such neglect of one eye can lead, most importantly, to the development of amblyopia — 'lazy eye'. This, in turn, if allowed to persist beyond the age of about 7 years, will be irreversible, with impairment of vision.

The main causes of squint in childhood are:

— Heredity
— High degrees of refractive error
— Ocular disease, preventing the proper development of vision.

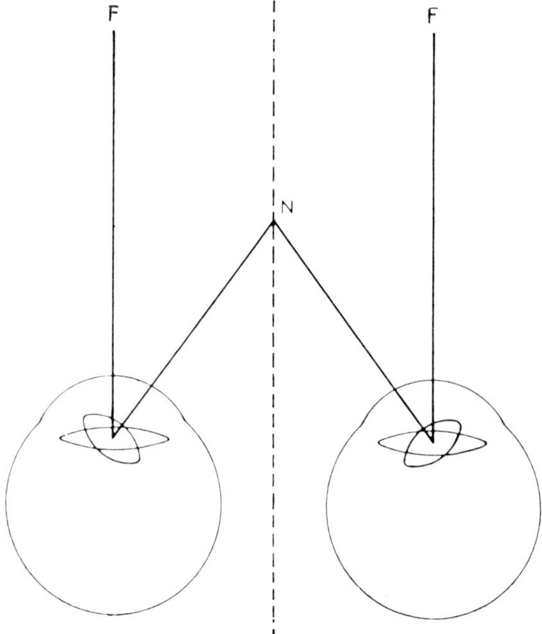

Fig. 12.1 The Accommodation–Convergence Relationship. If the eyes are considered, in the first instance, as regarding a distant object (F) a clear retinal image is obtained in each eye without any effort of either accommodation or convergence. On looking at a near object (N) a balanced relationship normally exists between the degree of accommodation exerted and the angle of convergence. In hypermetropia this relationship is upset.

Errors of refraction and squint

To look at a close object, it is necessary not only to focus the eyes by the use of accommodation but also to exercise convergence.

In hypermetropia, the amount of accommodation is out of proportion to the amount of convergence needed at a given distance (Fig. 12.1), and the child may not be able to dissociate these functions, with resultant over-convergence.

Ocular disease and squint

If any ocular disorder prevents the proper development of binocular vision, a squint may result. In addition to refractive errors, possible causes are corneal opacities, cataract, retinal disease and optic atrophy. Clinical varieties of concomitant squint:

— Convergent (esotropia)/divergent (exotropia)
— Constant/intermittent
— Uniocular/alternating.

Presentation

Although occasionally present at birth, the onset of a squint is typically around 3 years of age. The deviation, intermittent at first, is often noticed by someone other than the parents, and is more obvious when the child is tired, angry or unwell.

A child does not 'grow out of' a squint, and time spent waiting for spontaneous cure is time wasted.

Diagnosis

The commonest cause of a mistaken diagnosis of squint is epicanthus, making the cornea seem closer to the midline than it actually is (Fig. 12.2). If in any doubt, the relative positions of the bright reflexes from the cornea must be assessed. If the eyes are 'straight' the bright reflection of a torch will be symmetrical in the two eyes.

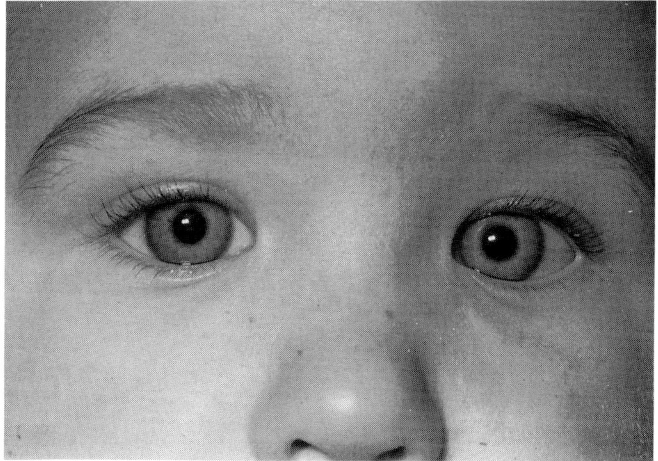

Fig. 12.2 Epicanthus

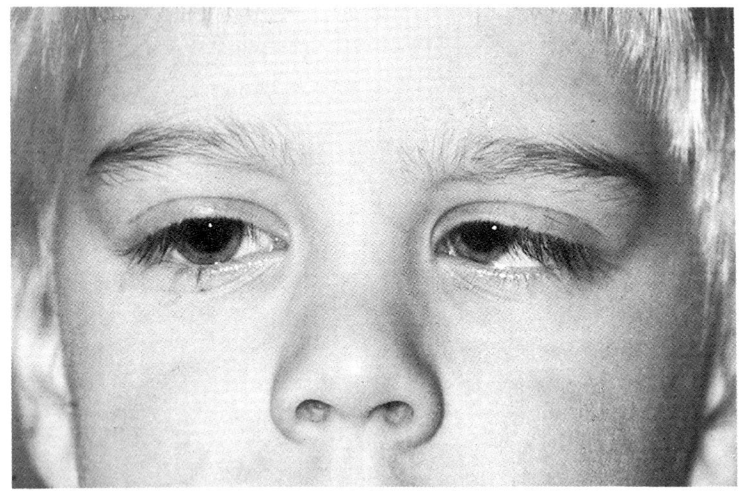

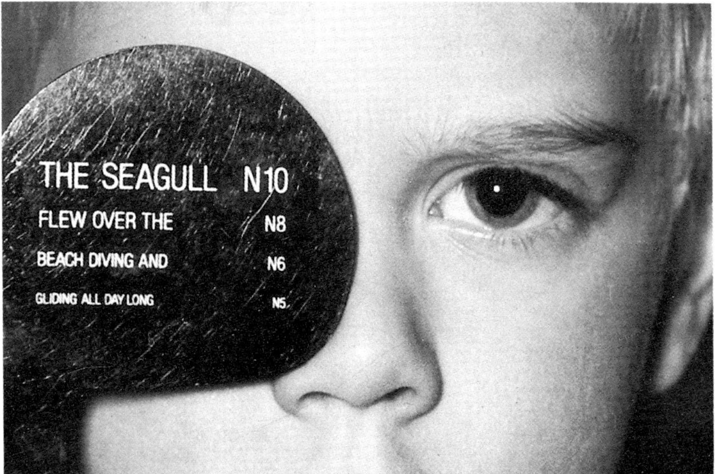

Fig. 12.3 The cover test: left convergent squint.

The other invaluable test is the cover test (Fig. 12.3). Ensuring that the child's attention is attracted, the eyes are covered in turn. If each eye remains stationary when the fellow eye is covered, no squint is present. If, however, on covering one eye, the opposite eye moves to take up fixation, that eye was originally squinting.

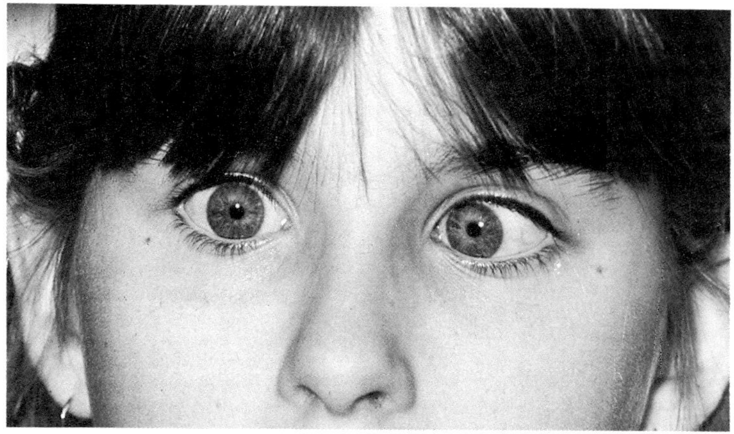

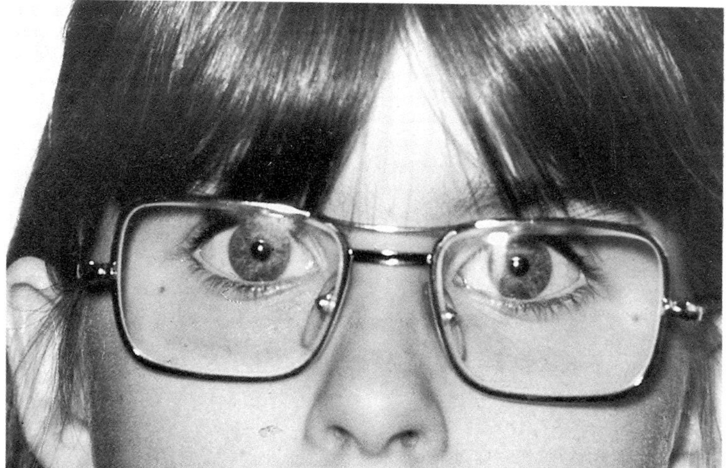

Fig. 12.4 Accommodative convergent squint, controlled with spectacles.

Treatment

The treatment of squint consists of the following steps, the detailed application of which will be decided by the ophthalmologist:

1. *Refraction*, providing spectacles if indicated (Fig. 12.4), and fundus examination.

2. *Occlusion of the fixing eye*, to force the amblyopic eye into activity.

3. *Orthoptic supervision*, to assess the state of binocular vision and to assist in the planning of surgery.

4. *Operation* may be required in the treatment of those who do not respond to the provision of glasses together with orthoptic treatment. Adjustment of the visual axes is achieved by planned weakening (recession) of the overactive muscles, combined with strengthening (advancement or resection) of the antagonists. The extent of the surgery is largely based on measurements obtained in the orthoptic department.

Surgery is the only possible treatment in neglected cases showing incurable amblyopia, when the problem is purely cosmetic. General anaesthesia is usual, but the hospital stay is short; the child goes home as soon as he has fully recovered from the anaesthetic.

Divergent squint (exotropia)

This condition is less common than convergent squint. It presents at a later age and is usually seen on distant gaze. The child may be noticed to close one eye in bright light.

Treatment is surgical and the prognosis good. Operation is generally advised if the squint is present more then 50% of the time or is cosmetically unsatisfactory. Older children with intermittent diplopia associated with a divergent squint may also require surgery.

Latent squint (heterophoria)

In adults, a state of imbalance between the muscles of the two eyes, not sufficient to lead to actual squint, can lead to symptoms of eyestrain, particularly on reading. A well-defined cause of this difficulty is 'convergence insufficiency'. As is the case in various types of heterophoria, convergence insufficiency often responds to treatment by an orthoptist.

Paralytic squint

Usually seen in later life, these squints may be due to trauma, intracranial vascular accidents, aneurysms, tumours, and multiple sclerosis.

Symptoms

The only symptom is diplopia, often leading to giddiness and nausea, and usually worse in one direction of the gaze.

Diagnosis

A marked squint may be obvious, or there may be evident limitation of movement of an eye.

The cause usually lies within the central nervous system. Most paralytic squints occurring in the elderly recover in a few weeks and are due to small arteriosclerotic lesions.

Third nerve palsy: Complete oculomotor paralysis gives ptosis, a dilated, unreacting pupil with a normal consensual response in the other eye to a stimulus in the affected eye, and deviation of the paralysed eye laterally and downwards. This is due to the unopposed actions of the superior oblique and lateral rectus muscles.

Usually, oculomotor nerve lesions are incomplete. A third nerve palsy sparing the pupil is likely to be due to the vascular complications of diabetes.

Fourth nerve palsy: Trochlear nerve palsy is less common than lesions of the third and sixth nerves. The patient may adopt a compensatory head posture due to the vertical and torsional actions of the superior oblique muscle. The difficulty is in looking down and in reading.

Bilateral superior oblique palsy is usually due to head injury.

Sixth nerve palsy: Weakness of the lateral rectus muscle produces defective abduction of the eye. The patient may adopt a head turn toward the opposite side to minimize diplopia.

Analysis of paralytic squint

The patient is asked to follow the movement of a hand in the various directions of the gaze, as indicated, and the position of maximum separation of the images is determined. The eyes are then covered in turn, demonstrating which image is furthest displaced. The 'furthest away' image belongs to the eye with the paralysed muscle. (Fig. 12.5)

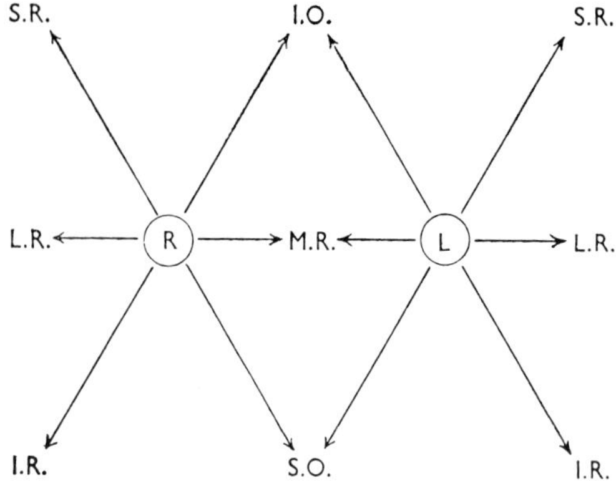

Fig. 12.5 Analysis of paralytic squint.

Management

The need to investigate patients with paralytic squint of recent onset depends on the age at presentation and on whether there are other neurological abnormalities. Referral is always appropriate, though if the lesion is arteriosclerotic, recovery is usual within a few weeks.

While awaiting recovery, a temporary prism attached to the glasses, or an injection of botulinum toxin into the antagonist muscle, may be helpful. If recovery fails to occur, surgery may be indicated to restore an effective, if not a complete, field of binocular vision.

Patients with paralytic diplopia should not drive. A paralytic squint in an older, arteriosclerotic patient should be regarded as a minor stroke and may be the forerunner of a major cerebrovascular accident.

Myasthenia gravis may present with ptosis (p. 25) or weakness of extraocular muscles leading to diplopia. Diagnosis is confirmed by a positive Tensilon® test and by the demonstration of motor endplate receptor antibodies in a blood sample.

Gaze palsy

Interference with the supranuclear control of eye movements leads to limitation of gaze in one or more directions. The cause may be multiple sclerosis, Parkinson's disease, a vascular lesion or a tumour. A neurologist's advice should be sought.

Internuclear ophthalmoplegia

Failure of either eye to adduct on lateral gaze, with nystagmus of the abducting eye, is due to a lesion in the medial longitudinal bundle. Internuclear ophthalmoplegia is not uncommon in multiple sclerosis.

NYSTAGMUS

Nystagmus — involuntary, oscillatory movements of the eyes — is either jerky, with fast and slow components, or pendular. The cause may be in the labyrinthine or visual systems.

Jerky nystagmus is seen under certain circumstances in normal individuals. Examples in the vestibular system are the induction of nystagmus on caloric stimulation of the ears and on rotation of the head. In the visual system, optokinetic nystagmus occurs when objects are fixated in rapid succession, as when looking through the window of a moving train, and in 'end point' nystagmus the eyes oscillate on extreme lateral gaze.

Vestibular nystagmus occurs in disorders of the middle ear and its central connections, and of the cerebellum. The movements are jerky, with the fast component toward the side of the lesion. Pendular nystagmus is seen in children whose vision has been markedly impaired in both eyes since birth, or becomes so during the first year or two of life. It arises because the normal fixation reflexes cannot become established.

Congenital nystagmus is a fairly common inherited condition. The movements are horizontal, vertical or rotatory. Usually there is one position of gaze in which they are least marked, and the patient may adopt a compensatory head posture so that the eyes assume this position, thereby obtaining optimum vision. Corrective surgery or prismatic lenses sometimes help.

In the absence of other ocular disorders, most children with congenital nystagmus achieve good near vision, so they can read small print and cope with normal schooling, but their distance vision is generally not better than 6/18 (Snellen). Hence parents should be warned that their child may not have good enough vision to be eligible for a driving licence (Ch. 17). This may have important consequences for employment.

Surgery has a place in the management of some cases in which a compensatory head posture is adopted.

Latent nystagmus

Latent nystagmus is not apparent when both eyes are fixing, but becomes manifest when either eye is covered. The condition is of no importance clinically unless the sight in one eye is unfortunately lost; but it may be the cause of failure when each eye is tested separately. When tested with both eyes in use, vision is normal.

AMBLYOPIA (Lazy eye)

Defined as reduced acuity in an eye without detectable disorder of the retina or visual pathways, amblyopia due to squint has been considered on page 123. Other causes are stimulus deprivation, as in ptosis or congenital cataract, in which the defect must be corrected as early as possible if useful vision is to be achieved, and unequal refractive errors in the two eyes (anisometropia). A difference in hypermetropia greater than 1 dioptre, or in myopia greater than 3 dioptres, may lead to amblyopia in the absence of a squint. Provided the refractive difference is not excessive, optical correction combined with occlusion of the eye with normal vision usually gives markedly improved, if not normal, acuity in the amblyopic eye. Best results are obtained under 6 or 7 years of age, but limited improvement may be obtained in older children. Inadequately corrected astigmatism may lead to partial amblyopia in both eyes.

Slight amblyopia, with reduced acuity when measured by reading Snellen test type lines, may escape detection with single letter-matching tests like the Sheridan Gardiner (p. 5). This phenomenon, known as 'crowding', should be borne in mind when interpreting the results of letter-matching tests.

13. Glaucoma

Any condition in which intraocular pressure is raised, with damage to vision, is glaucoma. 21 mmHg is considered to be the upper limit of normal.

Aqueous humour is produced by the ciliary body and passes through the pupil to the anterior chamber, leaving through pores in the trabecular meshwork, and entering the canal of Schlemm — an encircling channel at the corneoscleral junction — returning to the blood stream via the episcleral plexus of veins.

Glaucoma is classified according its cause, and may be primary or secondary (Table 13.1).

Table 13.1 Classification of glaucoma

Primary glaucoma	Secondary glaucoma
Congenital	Post-traumatic
Primary angle-closure	Uveitis
Primary open-angle	Lens-induced
	Thrombotic
	Steroids
	(Others)

CONGENITAL GLAUCOMA (Buphthalmos)

Occasionally present at birth, this condition is so rare that a general practitioner is unlikely to see it, but early recognition is essential for successful treatment.

Congenital abnormalities in the trabecular meshwork impede the drainage of aqueous. The infant's eyes water profusely and are red and painful. Attacks of pain may be intermittent in the early stages. The cornea has a ground glass appearance and becomes enlarged beyond the normal diameter of 10.5 mm. There may be splits in the deeper layers of the cornea. The globe enlarges and the optic disc becomes cupped. Any suspected case must be referred urgently. Treatment is surgical.

PRIMARY ANGLE-CLOSURE GLAUCOMA (Acute, congestive glaucoma)

Acute glaucoma is one of the emergencies of ophthalmology; it is rare below the age of 60. A general practitioner is unlikely to see more than one acute case in his lifetime.

Pathogenesis

Gradual shallowing of the anterior chamber as the lens enlarges with age predisposes to angle closure; it cannot develop in eyes with deep anterior chambers (Fig. 13.1). The intraocular pressure rises — usually suddenly. The pupil becomes fixed in mid-dilatation and, with increasing pressure, corneal oedema occurs.

The condition may also develop insidiously. Such cases are differentiated from open-angle glaucoma by detailed examination with a special contact lens (gonioscopy).

Presentation

Typically, the patient complains of sudden onset of pain with blurred vision (usually down to 'counting fingers' or 'hand movements'). One eye is affected, but the stress resulting from the attack may precipitate a similar situation in the other eye. Collapse and vomiting may occur if the pain is severe.

The eye is red, with corneal oedema preventing a clear view of iris detail, and the pupil is fixed and semi-dilated (Fig. 13.2). Raised intraocular pressure is obvious on palpation of the eye through the closed lids: the eye feels stony hard.

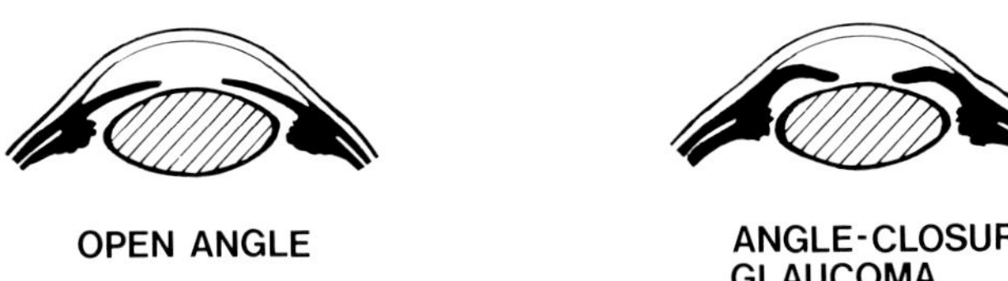

Fig. 13.1 Diagram of open and narrow angles

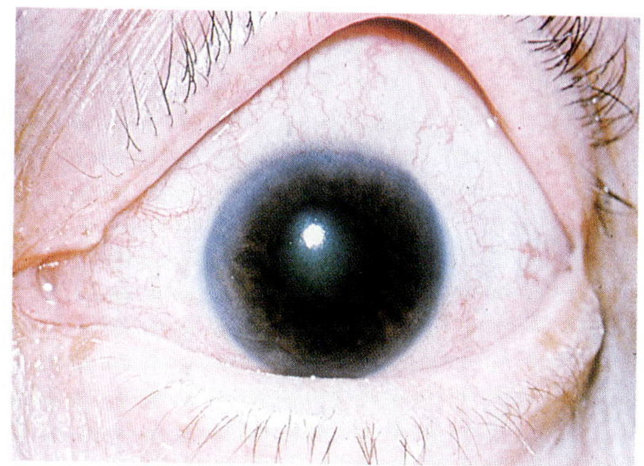

Fig. 13.2 Acute glaucoma

There may be a history of previous visual disturbance, particularly of seeing coloured haloes round white lights in the evening, perhaps with pain and blurring. These attacks may initially be self-limiting and relieved by sleep, during which the pupil normally contracts. Such a history requires referral as a glaucoma suspect, even without evidence of established angle closure.

The use of mydriatic drops to dilate the pupil for examination of the fundus — for example in the routine review of diabetics — may, very rarely, precipitate an attack of angle closure. In eyes seen to have shallow anterior chambers, demonstrable by shining a light obliquely on to the cornea and finding only part of the convex iris illuminated, these drops should be used with caution.

Management

All cases must be referred as emergencies. Hospital treatment is with intensive pilocarpine drops — usually 4% instilled every minute for 5 min, and every 5 min for half an hour — and intravenous acetazolamide (Diamox®) 500 mg. Additional medical treatment may be necessary and 2% pilocarpine is used prophylactically in the fellow eye. Definitive treatment is surgical — making a hole in the peripheral iris to permit the passage of aqueous into the anterior chamber, by-passing the pupil. This may be achieved either by laser iridotomy or peripheral iridectomy. Provided that permanent damage has not occurred in the drainage angle by adhesion formation, the patient is then cured. The fellow eye usually requires prophylactic operation.

PRIMARY OPEN-ANGLE GLAUCOMA (Chronic simple glaucoma)

A common and still incompletely understood condition, open-angle glaucoma occurs in about 2% of people over age 40, with increasing incidence in older age groups. It is bilateral and a common cause of blindness: early diagnosis gives the best chance of satisfactory treatment. Family history is of great importance — the incidence in first-degree relatives of glaucoma sufferers is several times higher than in the normal population. Siblings and children of patients with glaucoma are particularly at risk.

Pathogenesis

Drainage of aqueous at the trabecular meshwork is impeded, despite free access to the angle, for reasons that are not clear. The consequence is raised intraocular pressure, resulting in damage to the disc. This leads to characteristic atrophy of the nerve fibres at the optic disc (cupping) (Fig. 13.3) and visual field defects which, if the pressure is not controlled, progress to blindness.

It is common to find raised intraocular pressure without disc changes or field loss — termed 'ocular hypertension'.

Treatment is not required, but regular review of the condition is mandatory. Routine monitoring of the state of the optic discs, together with careful and repeated examination of the field of vision, may be expected to disclose the early changes which would indicate the need for treatment.

Steroid eye preparations cause a rise in intraocular pressure in susceptible individuals if used for more than a few weeks. Pressure checks are therefore necessary. If increased pressure is found and the continued use of steroid is considered essential, the ophthalmologist may decide to use one of the available steroids which are less prone to this side effect — fluorometholone (FML®) or clobetasone (Eumovate®).

Risk factors in open-angle glaucoma, apart from increasing with age over 40 and with a family history, have been identified as high myopia, diabetes, ischaemic heart disease and a history of a bleeding episode requiring blood transfusion.

Diagnosis

Most cases are detected in the course of routine sight tests. Several surveys in the United Kingdom have shown that general prac-

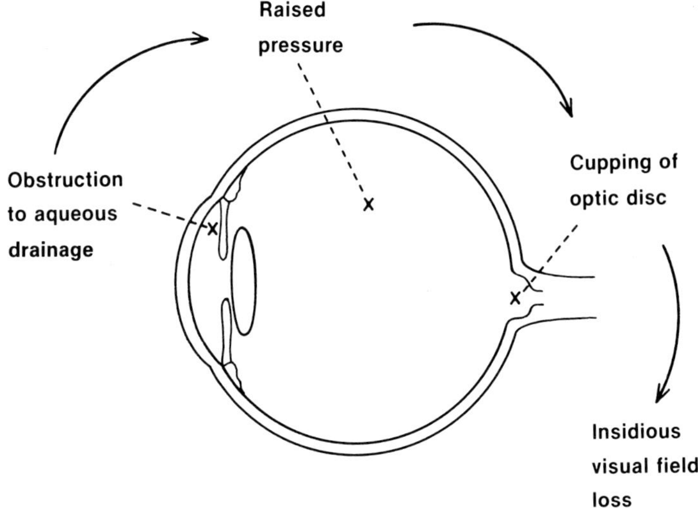

Fig. 13.3

titioners had suspected the diagnosis in about 5% of patients referred to eye clinics and found to have glaucoma. The factors taken into account in making the diagnosis are:

— Cupping of the disc
— Raised intraocular pressure
— Visual field loss.

Cupping of the disc

This is the feature most accessible to the general practitioner and every opportunity should be taken to practise the assessment of discs for possible glaucomatous changes. All doubtful cases, as well as those with apparently obvious changes, should be referred for further assessment. In this way the general practitioner's share of glaucoma referrals will increase! But it is not easy; even experts find it impossible to distinguish normal from glaucomatous discs with certainty.

The feature to look for particularly is the uniformity of width of the disc margin and symmetry in both eyes. Note should also be taken of:

1. *The size of the cup,* expressed as cup–disc ratio. 1.0 indicates complete cupping and 0.5 that the cup extends for half the overall

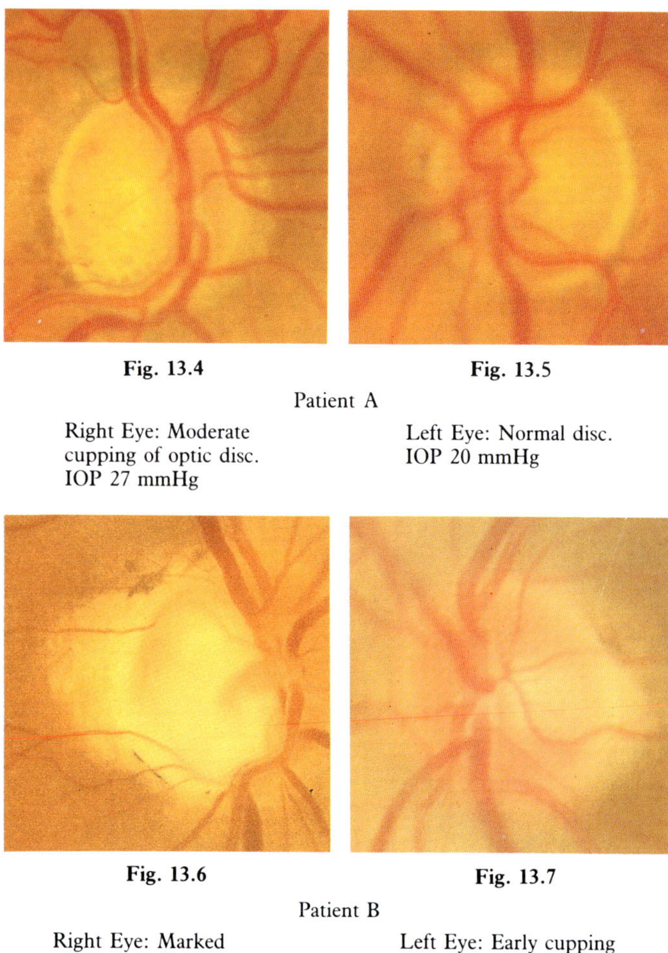

Fig. 13.4

Fig. 13.5

Patient A

Right Eye: Moderate cupping of optic disc. IOP 27 mmHg

Left Eye: Normal disc. IOP 20 mmHg

Fig. 13.6

Fig. 13.7

Patient B

Right Eye: Marked cupping of disc. Loss of upper field. IOP 31 mmHg

Left Eye: Early cupping of disc. Virtually full field. IOP 25 mmHg

disc diameter. 'Physiological' cupping is seen in healthy eyes, but a high cup–disc ratio carries a strong suspicion of glaucoma.

2. *A vertically oval cup* (vertical cup–disc ratio greater than horizontal) usually correlates with glaucomatous field loss.

3. *Asymmetry* between the disc cupping in the two eyes frequently suggests glaucoma.

4. *Haemorrhage* at the disc margin, suggesting circulatory embarrassment at the optic nerve head, makes a diagnosis of glaucoma likely.

5. *Pallor* of the disc is more difficult to evaluate: it may be of significance, but cupping is a more reliable sign. Advanced cases of glaucoma always have pale discs (Figs 13.4–13.7).

Fundus examination showing extensive retinal haemorrhages due to retinal vein occlusion (p. 86) indicates immediate referral. A venous occlusion may be the presenting feature of glaucoma.

Raised intraocular pressure

There are as many pitfalls in intraocular pressure measurement and the conclusions drawn from it as from disc assessment. Guessing the pressure from palpation of the globe is useless, except in the extreme case of acute angle-closure glaucoma (p. 134).

It is by no means incumbent on general practitioners to measure intraocular pressure (tonometry), but if a doctor or his practice assistants are to do so, two suitable instruments are available. The Perkins® hand-held tonometer (Fig. 13.8) is portable and accurate; considerable practice is required to achieve proficiency in its use. More expensive, but rather easier to use, and of comparable accuracy, is the Keeler 'Pulsair' Tonometer® (Fig. 13.9). It has the advantage of being 'non-contact', so neither anaesthetic drops or sterilization are required. The increasing incidence of open-angle glaucoma over age 40 makes tonometry a valuable screening procedure in routine medical checks.

Routine tonometry is usually carried out in the course of eye examination for refraction. Patients found at refraction to have intraocular pressures over 21 mmHg are commonly referred to the general practitioner. It helps the ophthalmologist considerably if the referral letter is accompanied by all the details given on the report, together with relevant medical information, particularly with regard to respiratory and cardiovascular disorders.

Visual field examination

To detect glaucomatous loss at an early stage is time consuming and may require complex apparatus. This aspect of diagnosis is therefore outside the scope of general practice.

Once field loss is sufficiently advanced to attract the patient's attention, the glaucoma is likely to be far advanced. Early diagnosis is the key to successful management.

Glaucomatous field loss tends to be more severe in patients with

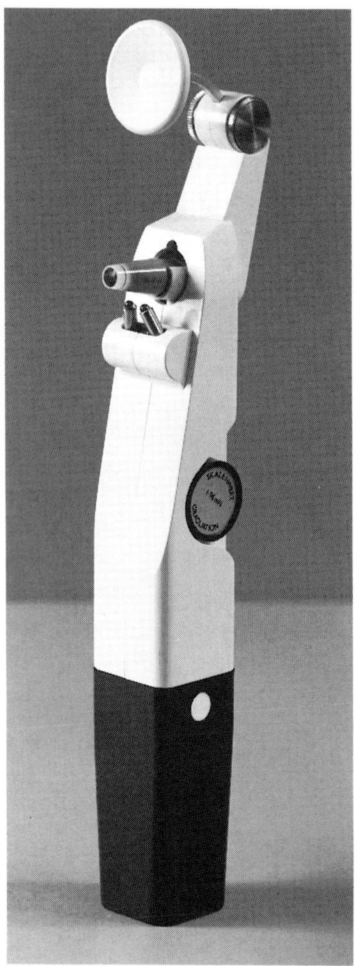

Fig. 13.8 Perkins applanation tonometer Mk 2. No filter sleeves fitted.

generalized arteriosclerosis, due, probably, to poor perfusion at the optic nerve head. Sudden exacerbation of field loss may be seen after acute illnesses such as coronary thrombosis, severe gastrointestinal haemorrhage or major surgery in which there has been a period of significantly lowered blood pressure.

Field loss and disc cupping without raised intraocular pressure represent damage to the disc without impaired drainage of aqueous.

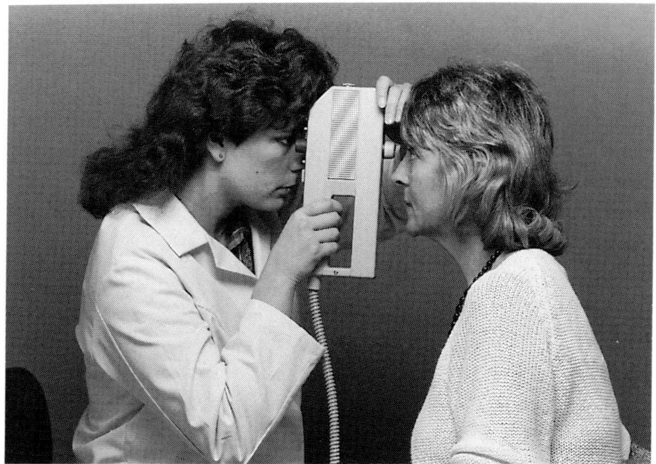

Fig. 13.9 Keeler Pulse-Air tonometer

This condition is termed 'low-tension glaucoma'. Treatment is difficult.

Management

All suspected cases of glaucoma should be referred. Priority should be indicated. It is preferable that treatment be withheld until after the first consultation with the specialist in order that a true baseline assessment can be made.

Raised pressure alone, without disc or field changes ('ocular hypertension') requires specialist follow-up but is not usually treated. If there is any evidence of change in the disc appearance or visual field loss, treatment for glaucoma must be given.

The choice is between drug therapy by eye drops (or, rarely, oral agents), conventional glaucoma drainage surgery and laser trabeculoplasty. It is usual to try drug therapy with drops initially. The other means are reserved for those who do not respond satisfactorily, due either to failure to tolerate the regime or to its ineffectiveness, manifested by persistently raised pressure and progressive field loss. However, a growing body of ophthalmic opinion favours immediate laser trabeculoplasty or surgical trabulectomy.

Medical

The drugs commonly used and their side effects are listed in Table 13.2. Most frequently prescribed are topical beta-blockers and pilocarpine 0.5 to 4.0%. Pilocarpine is also available as slow-release 'Ocuserts®' which are inserted into the lower conjunctival fornix and changed weekly.

Patient 'compliance' is all-important, and it is the responsibility of the ophthalmologist, supported by the general practitioner, to ensure that the patient understands why glaucoma drugs have been prescribed and that their aim is the preservation of useful sight, rather than the improvement of vision.

The general practitioner should be aware of the potentially dangerous side effects of beta-blockers (Table 13.2). If in doubt, stop the drug and refer.

Surgical

Patients in whom glaucoma is not adequately controlled by medical treatment require surgery to bring the pressure to 21 mmHg or less and prevent further field loss. The surgical procedure most commonly used is trabeculectomy, in which a small block of tissue is removed from the trabecular meshwork. A drainage 'bleb' or blister usually results and can be seen behind the limbus under the upper lid.

The operation may be done under general or local anaesthesia. Accelerated cataract formation is a disadvantage of glaucoma surgery.

An alternative and increasingly popular treatment is laser trabeculoplasty. Up to 100 small burns are applied with an argon laser to the trabecular meshwork. This is an out-patient procedure without significant complications. It appears to be successful in many cases.

Treatment by conventional drainage surgery or laser trabeculoplasty may free patients from the need to take regular medication, but most are advised to have periodic checks to ensure than the glaucoma remains satisfactorily controlled.

Glaucoma requires a lifetime of regular ophthalmic supervision and the general practitioner may be asked to make inquiries of defaulters. He also has a role in advising relatives of glaucoma patients, who are at risk, to seek appropriate examination.

Table 13.2 Drugs commonly used in open-angle glaucoma

Group	Non-proprietory name	Proprietory name	Inconvenient side effects	Serious side effects
β-adrenergic antagonists (β-blockers)	Betaxolol 0.5% twice daily* Carteolol 1–2% twice daily Levobunolol 0.5% once or twice daily Metipranolol 0.1–0.5% twice daily Timolol 0.25–0.5% twice daily	Betoptic Teoptic Betagan Glauline Timoptol	Local irritation	Bronchospasm, worsening of asthma and of chronic lung disease, bradycardia, dangerous in heart block
Miotics (parasympathomimetics)	Pilocarpine 0.5–4.0% up to 4 times daily	Isopto Carpine Ocusert Sno Pilo	Brow ache, small pupil, transient myopia, gastrointestinal spasm	
Sympathomimetics	Adrenaline 0.5–1% twice daily Dipivefrin hydrochloride 0.1% twice daily	Eppy Simplene Epiphrin Propine	Local irritation Red eyes Tachycardia	Angle closure with narrow angles Cystoid macular oedema in aphakia
Carbonic anhydrase inhibitors	Acetazolamide 0.5 to 1 g daily Dichlorphenamide 100–200 mg daily	Diamox Daranide	Gastrointestinal disturbance Paraesthesiae	Blood dyscrasias, electrolyte imbalance, gastrointestinal irritation, urinary calculi, weight loss

Note *betaxolol is a cardioselective β_1-antagonist and less likely to produce bronchoconstriction.

SECONDARY GLAUCOMA

Uveitis

Iritis or iridocyclitis may be accompanied by raised intraocular pressure, usually settling as the inflammation subsides. Drugs to reduce intraocular pressure may be needed in addition to those prescribed to control the uveitis (see p. 66).

Lens-induced glaucoma

A hypermature cataract, seen as a white opacity in the pupil, may degenerate and obstruct aqueous drainage by the collection of material in the trabeculum, or swell and cause angle-closure glaucoma. Any patient with a red painful eye and a dense, mature cataract should be referred urgently.

Post-traumatic glaucoma

Blunt injury, usually causing hyphaema (p. 103) originally, may predispose to glaucoma by damaging the drainage angle. This accounts for a number of apparently unilateral cases of glaucoma. Patients who have sustained significant injury to an eye should be watched with more than usual vigilance for glaucoma and should report the history of injury when undergoing routine eye tests.

Thrombotic glaucoma

Associated with rubeosis iridis (common causes: proliferative diabetic retinopathy and central retinal vein occlusion with ischaemia), this presents as pain in a blind eye (see p. 86). New vessels are visible on the surface of the iris. Treatment is unsatisfactory.

Drugs

The use of steroid drops or ointment in or around the eye for periods longer than a week or two leads to raised intraocular pressure in susceptible individuals (see p. 136).

14. The visual pathway

OPTIC NERVE

The general practitioner can inspect the optic nerve at the optic disc, and can assess its function by testing pupil reactions (p. 7), visual acuity, colour vision and visual fields. Complex equipment is needed to test function electrically (see Ch. 16).

Congenital abnormalities

A number of congenital abnormalities of the optic disc are recognized:

Myelinated nerve fibres (Fig. 14.1)
Drusen of the optic disc (Fig. 14.2)
Coloboma of the optic disc
Tilted optic disc
Optic disc hypoplasia
Optic disc pit.

Of these, drusen may mimic papilloedema; coloboma and tilting of the optic disc may be associated with visual field defects. About 30% of eyes with optic disc pits later develop macular oedema and failure of central vision. Optic disc hypoplasia may be a cause of poor vision.

Optic atrophy

Disorders of the optic nerve producing pallor of the optic disc (optic atrophy) are listed in Table 14.1.

1. *Trauma.* Usually a severe blow to the eye or side of the head. Apart from loss of vision, the only sign may be an afferent pupillary defect. Skull X-rays are advisable, but may show no fracture. Optic atrophy develops in 6–8 weeks.

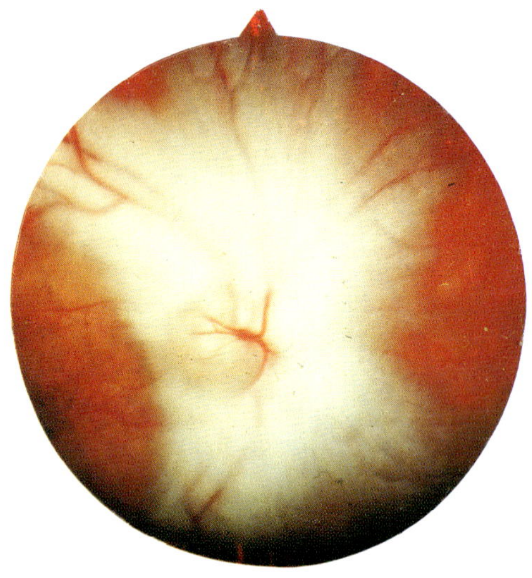

Fig. 14.1 Myelinated nerve fibres

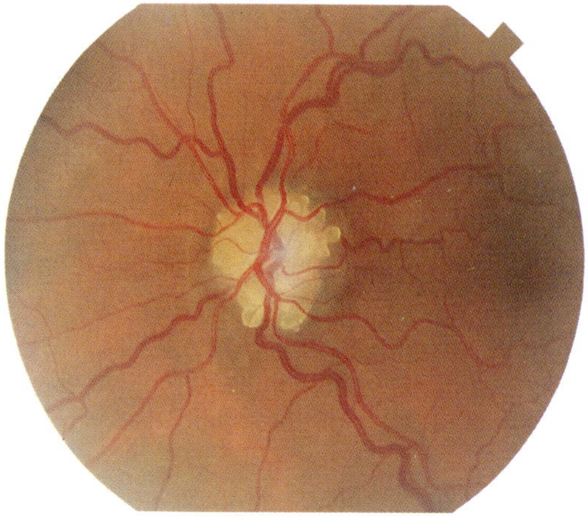

Fig. 14.2 Drusen of optic disc

2. *Ischaemia of the retina*. Occlusion of the central retinal artery is followed some weeks later by optic atrophy (see p. 84).

3. *Ischaemia of the optic nerve* has two common causes:

Giant cell arteritis. Perhaps the most important ophthalmic con-

Table 14.1 Causes of acquired optic atrophy

Trauma
Ischaemia — of the retina
Ischaemia — of the optic nerve
Compressive lesions of the visual pathway
Toxic or nutritional optic nerve damage
Glaucoma
Retinitis pigmentosa
Resolved papilloedema

dition encountered in general practice, arteritic ischaemic optic neuropathy is a medical emergency. It usually occurs over the age of 60. There may be prodromal symptoms of temporal arteritis — malaise, weight loss, pain on chewing, discomfort when wearing a hat, and headache. Sudden and profound loss of vision occurs and a pale swollen disc is seen with loss of direct pupillary reaction. Episodes of transient visual loss (amaurosis fugax) may have occurred previously.

The diagnosis is all but confirmed by finding a significantly raised ESR (usually over 50 mm/h) or plasma viscosity (usually over 1.9). Immediate treatment with high dosage steroid by mouth is essential: the usual starting dose is prednisolone 120 mg daily, reducing as the ESR falls.

The patient may be referred for a temporal artery biopsy, but treatment must come first. Failure to start early and adequate steroid therapy may result in the even more disastrous loss of vision in the second eye.

'Anterior' ischaemic optic neuropathy is the cumbersome term for a condition that affects the optic nerve head and is not accompanied by giant cell arteritis. The diagnosis can only be made when arteritis has been excluded (Fig. 14.3). The onset of visual loss is more gradual than in giant cell arteritis and may be less profound. The optic disc is swollen, often with associated flame-shaped haemorrhages and there is an afferent pupil defect. The ESR is normal.

Management. Having excluded giant cell arteritis, other factors predisposing to arterial occlusion should be sought — hypertension, diabetes and lipid disorders. There is less likelihood of bilateral involvement than in giant cell arteritis: prophylactic treatment with low dose aspirin may be advised.

4. *Optic neuritis* (Fig. 14.4b). Termed 'retrobulbar' neuritis if the swelling is sufficiently near the optic nerve head to cause disc swell-

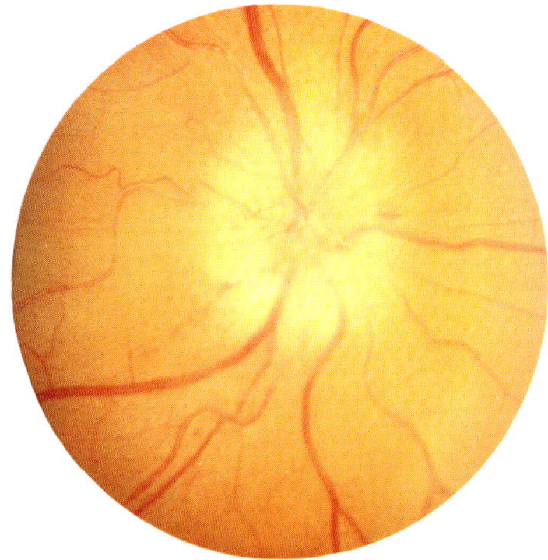

Fig. 14.3 Ischaemic optic neuropathy

ing, the onset is usually in the 20–45 age group, but children may be affected. The cause, like that of multiple sclerosis, is not known. There is a positive association with histocompatibility antigen HLA-DR2.

The patient complains of impaired vision — maybe as poor as mere perception of light. There is impaired colour discrimination (best shown with a red target) and a central visual field defect. The eye may be tender to the touch, with discomfort on looking to the side. The afferent pupillary defect is, in mild cases, an oscillating response to direct light. The swinging light test (p. 7) demonstrates impaired function in the affected optic nerve.

Optic nerve dysfunction can be quantified by testing visually evoked cortical responses, and demyelination in the optic nerve can be demonstrated by MRI scanning (see Ch. 16, electrodiagnostic tests).

Treatment does not affect the outcome of optic neuritis though ACTH or steroids may be recommended to speed recovery of vision. Most patients regain normal or near-normal vision after the first episode. More than 50% of previously healthy patients developing optic neuritis are found on follow-up to develop other symptoms of demyelinating disease, among which may be paralytic squint (q.v.). The exact proportion developing multiple sclerosis is uncertain, but some undoubtedly have no further neurological illness.

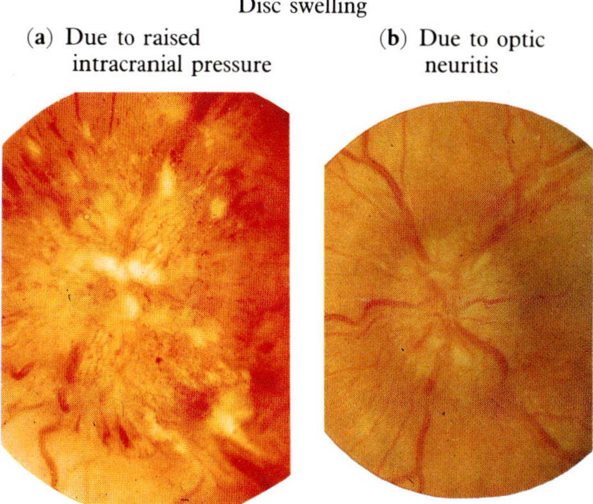

Fig. 14.4 Papilloedema

Certain drugs, particularly ethambutol, may cause optic neuritis.

5. *Compressive lesions of the optic nerve* are considered on page 150. Any patient with temporal visual field loss or unexplained loss of vision should raise suspicion of pituitary tumour or other compressive lesion. A lateral X-ray of the skull may show an enlarged pituitary fossa. Computerized tomography (CT) usually provides the diagnosis in chiasmal compression.

6. *Tobacco/alcohol optic neuropathy*. Older people who smoke, drink heavily and eat poorly are most at risk. Pipe smokers are predominant.

Presentation is with gradually decreasing visual acuity. Defective colour perception and a characteristic central visual field defect can be demonstrated. Both eyes are affected.

Treatment is by stopping smoking, withdrawing alcohol and giving multivitamins by mouth and hydroxycobalamine (Neocytamen®) by injection: 1000 μg daily for a week, weekly for a month and 3-monthly thereafter. The response to treatment is good.

7. *Glaucoma* — see page 139.

8. *Retinitis pigmentosa* — see page 99.

PAPILLOEDEMA (Fig. 14.4a)

Swelling of the optic disc may be due to papilloedema or pseudopapilloedema. The distinction may not be easy; all cases of doubt should be referred immediately.

Signs of papilloedema

Disc swelling
Haemorrhages near disc
Lack of pulsation of central retinal vein
Dilatation of retinal veins
Central visual acuity usually preserved.

Papilloedema is produced by a hold-up of the normal movement of axoplasm along the retinal nerve fibres into the optic nerve, leading to its accumulation at the optic disc. Among the causes are:

1. Raised intracranial pressure: usually with headaches, worse in the morning, and on straining. Vomiting and neurological localizing signs may occur.
2. Ischaemic optic neuropathy (p. 146).
3. Malignant hypertension (p. 83).
4. Optic neuritis (p. 147).

'Pseudo-papilloedema' refers to an optic disc which looks raised, but in which there is no obstruction to axoplasmic flow. The nerve fibres are functioning normally. The condition is seen in marked hypermetropia and, less often, when there are 'drusen' (hyaline-like, round deposits) within the optic nerve head (p. 146).

The distinction between true and pseudo-papilloedema is important and any case of doubt should be referred. Fluorescein angiography (p. 160) may be helpful in diagnosis.

INTERFERENCE WITH THE VISUAL PATHWAY

The eye may serve as a guide to the presence and location of intracranial disease by the finding of visual field changes: rough testing can be carried out by the confrontation method (p. 5).

Although the lesions producing visual field defects are multiple, the types of visual loss that they cause are characteristic (p. 153).

If the lesion is in front of the optic chiasm, the defect is strictly uniocular with an afferent pupillary defect demonstrable by the swinging light test (p. 7). The optic disc is pale and atrophic.

Lesions at the optic chiasm produce bitemporal hemianopia, due to interference with the crossing fibres which carry impulses from the nasal half of each retina. This is typical of pituitary tumours and the loss of field is usually asymmetrical (Fig. 14.5). Impaired colour recognition is an early sign.

Behind the chiasm any interference with the visual pathway

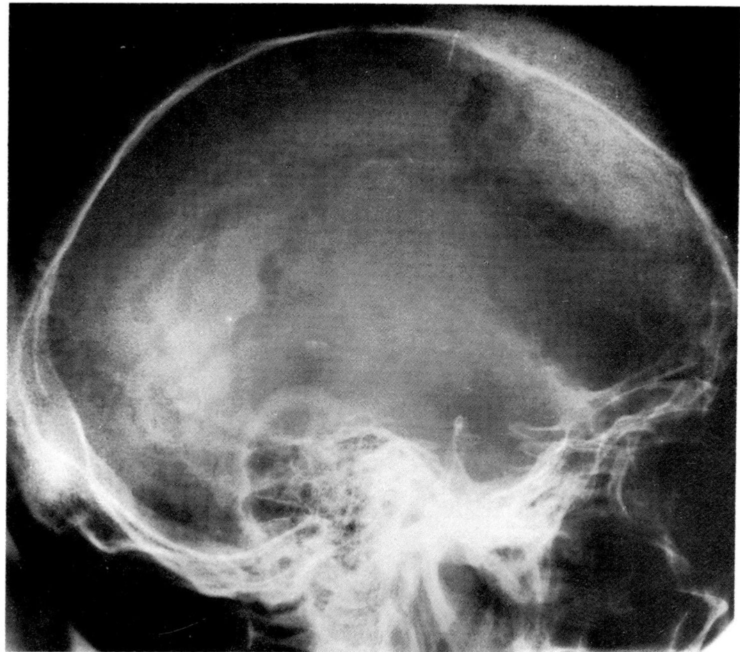

Fig. 14.5 Lateral radiograph of skull showing pituitary fossa enlarged by tumour. Note sloping 'double' floor of fossa and erosion of posterior clinoids.

(Fig. 14.6) will affect both eyes. The right optic tract, optic radiation and visual cortex receive impulses from the right halves of both retinae and damage here is projected into the left visual field. Similarly, the right visual field is served by the left visual pathway. A lesion behind the chiasm, therefore, leads to a homonymous field defect, lying in the same half of the field of vision of both eyes.

Running through the brain, with a synapse in the lateral geniculate nucleus, the fibres of the visual pathway terminate in the visual cortex at the occipital pole. They follow a consistent and well-defined pattern. Knowledge of the distribution of these fibres, combined with detailed analysis of visual field defects, allows accurate localization of a lesion.

Examples of typical visual field defects are given in Figure 14.7.

The results of visual field analysis together with the CT and MRI scans are invaluable in the investigation of intracranial disease.

By far the commonest cause of homonymous field loss is a stroke involving the optic radiation. This defect can be readily

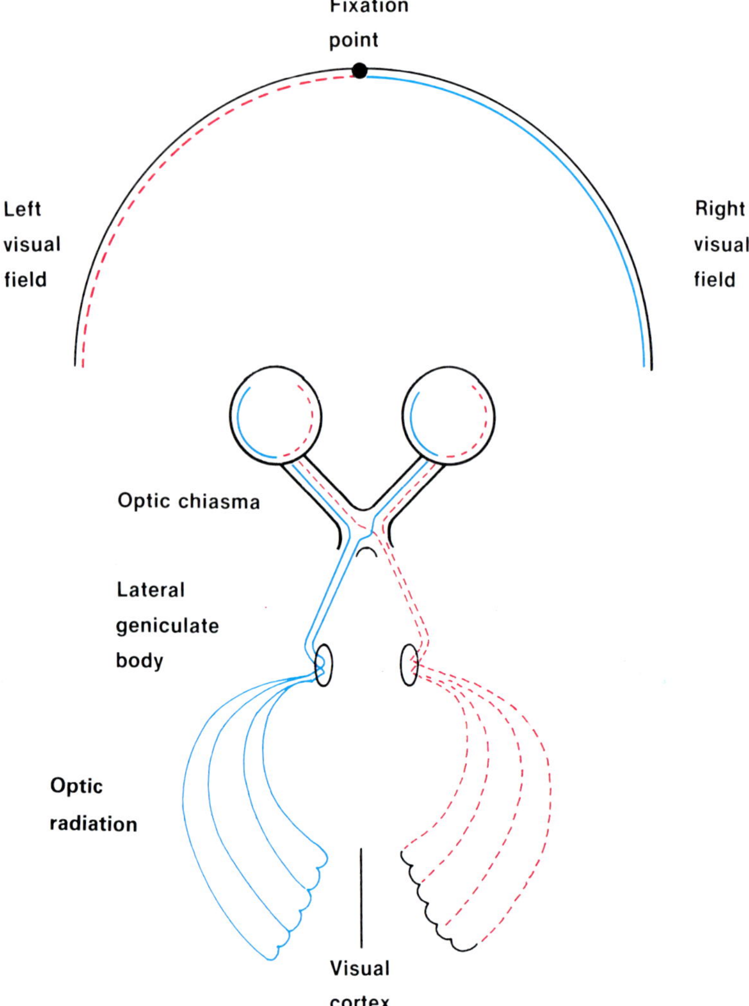

Fig. 14.6 The visual pathway

demonstrated by the general practitioner using the technique described on page 5.

MOTOR AND SENSORY LESIONS

In addition to producing visual field defects, intracranial lesions may interfere with ocular movements and produce sensory changes.

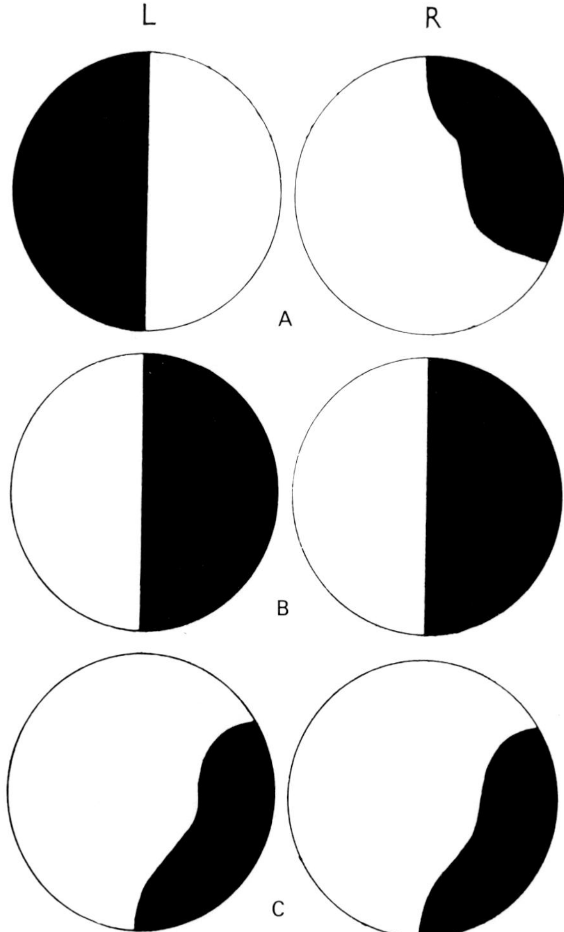

Fig. 14.7 Visual field changes, charted as seen by the patient.
(A) Bitemporal hemianopia. Pituitary lesion. Complete in the left eye. Incomplete in right.
(B) Homonymous hemianopia. Complete lesion of left visual pathway. Right-sided hemianopia.
(C) Incomplete homonymous hemianopia.

DISORDERS OF THE PUPIL

The technique for testing pupil reactions is described on page 7.

The following are some of the commoner pupillary abnormalities:

Tonic, or Holmes–Adie, pupil. The tonic pupil is semi-dilated and at first seems unreactive to light. If, however, the patient is exposed to bright light for some minutes, the pupil contracts slowly and dilates equally slowly on return to the dark. This occurs unilaterally in young people and is often associated with absence of deep tendon reflexes in the lower limbs. The condition is not associated with serious neurological disease.

Optic (retrobulbar) neuritis (see p. 147).

Horner's syndrome. The complete Horner's syndrome comprises a small pupil, ptosis, diminished sweating on the affected side of the face, and apparent enophthalmos. The condition is sometimes congenital but, if due to an active process, is caused by disease or injury affecting the sympathetic pathways.

The blind eye. In complete lesions of the optic nerve, perception of light is lost and with it the direct reaction of the pupil to light (afferent pupillary defect).

Accidental use of *mydriatic drugs* may occasionally be found unexpectedly.

Traumatic mydriasis. Direct injury to the eye may cause dilatation of the pupil (see p. 103).

Light–near dissociation. The pupil fails to react to light, but the near response persists. The causes include diabetes and disorders of the brain stem.

The Argyll Robertson pupils of neurosyphilis are small and irregular and react to a near stimulus while not reacting to light.

15. The orbit

Orbital disease usually presents as proptosis, the rigid walls of the orbit only allowing expansion of the contents anteriorly. Proptosis can most easily be seen when standing behind the seated patient. Measurement is carried out from the side, holding a ruler against the bony edge of the lateral wall of the orbit and estimating its distance from the apex of the cornea in profile. The two sides can be compared.

Double vision and displacement of the globe are also evidence of orbital disease.

Dysthyroid eye disease (Fig. 15.1)

The commonest orbital problem, proptosis may be unilateral or bilateral. CT scanning is indicated if the diagnosis is in doubt.

Other signs are:

1. *Lid retraction* — the superior corneal margin is visible: under normal circumstances the lid covers the upper third of the cornea.
2. *Lid lag* — the upper lid lags behind the eye in vertical movements.
3. *Double vision* — may result from involvement and tethering of the extraocular muscles.

The underlying cause of dysthyroid eye disease is not clear, but it may occur at any stage in the course of thyrotoxicosis and its treatment. Patients should be referred for ophthalmic assessment if complications prove a cosmetic embarrassment or a risk to sight. Hypothyroidism during the treatment of thyrotoxicosis may exacerbate eye complications and should be avoided.

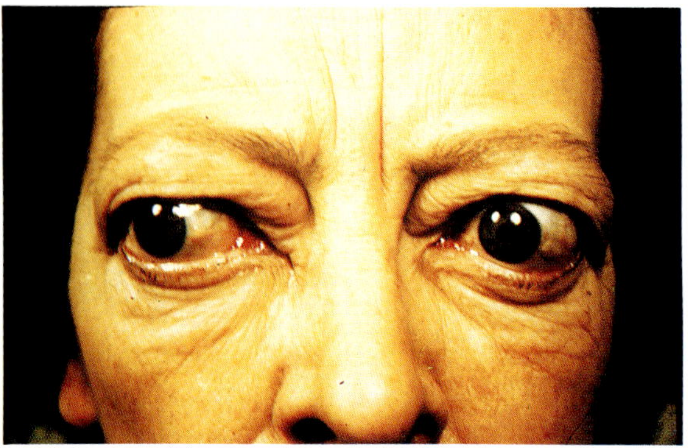

Fig. 15.1 Dysthyroid eye disease

Ophthalmic complications

1. Double vision
2. Exposure keratitis (see p. 60)
3. Retinal or optic nerve circulatory impairment and secondary glaucoma.

Threat to vision may necessitate treatment with high doses of steroid (120 mg prednisolone daily) or immunosuppressive drugs; more than half the patients respond. Surgical decompression of the orbit may be required.

In the event of the eyes failing to close properly in sleep, with risk of corneal exposure, taping the lids together at night is often helpful.

Dysthyroid eye disease is usually self-limiting. Most cases return to nearly normal appearance eventually, though the condition may persist for several years.

Orbital cellulitis

Infection of the orbital contents leads to painful proptosis, difficulty opening the eye, and redness of the skin. There is usually purulent discharge.

The commonest cause is sinus infection, usually ethmoiditis. Confirm by X-ray. Skin infections, injuries, and metastatic infection may occasionally cause orbital cellulitis.

Management should be in hospital. Drainage of pus from the

orbit or sinuses may be needed in addition to intensive antibiotic treatment.

Orbital tumours

Proptosis may be due to a tumour. If the displacement is axial, the tumour is likely to be within the cone of extraocular muscles. CT scanning is of great value in diagnosis.

Caroticocavernous fistula

Causes proptosis with engorged collateral blood vessels and pulsation of the globe. An orbital bruit may be heard. The patients are elderly.

Trauma

Blunt injury of the orbit may cause a 'blow-out' fracture. There is enophthalmos, limitation of gaze (usually upwards), and diplopia (see p. 107).

16. Special investigations in ophthalmology

The general practitioner will be notified of special investigations carried out on his patients. He may be asked by the patient for more information about the tests and for advice on their outcome.

Investigation of the lacrimal system

The simplest test of lacrimal drainage, apart from clinical examination and pressure over the sac to demonstrate retained contents, is syringing of the tear passage. Further information may be derived from radiography following injection of contrast medium into the canaliculus, and from lacrimal scintigraphy, in which a drop of short-lived radio-isotope is instilled into the conjunctival sac and its passage followed by gamma detector. The level and extent of obstruction are thus determined and treatment planned accordingly.

Electrodiagnosis

Three tests are commonly used:

1. *Electroretinogram* — the potential generated in the retina in response to a light stimulus is detected by two electrodes, one placed on the lower eyelid and the second on the forehead. The response is diminished or abolished in disorders of the retina such as retinitis pigmentosa.
2. *Electro-oculogram* — A mass electrical response is detected by electrodes, placed on the skin at the inner and outer corners of the eye, when the gaze is directed to either side. The response is reduced or abolished in disorders of the retinal pigment epithelium.
3. *Visually evoked cortical responses* — electrodes at the occiput detect activity in the underlying visual cortex in a manner simi-

lar to electroencephalography. A flash of light, or an alternating checkerboard at which the subject gazes, produces a response of which the timing and intensity can be measured.

The integrity of the pathway to the visual cortex can be verified in uncooperative subjects and in children. Delay in the passage of the impulse from one or both eyes indicates impaired conduction in the optic nerve as, for example, in demyelination.

Dark adaptometry

Assessment of the changing threshold during dark adaptation gives an index of rod and cone function.

Perimetry (visual field analysis)

Many devices are available for the analysis of visual fields. 'Static' perimetry involves the use of immobile stimuli of varying intensity; 'dynamic' perimetry denotes a stimulus of constant intensity which is moved across the visual fields to determine the thresholds.

These two methods are used to detect glaucomatous field loss and other defects which may be due to neurological or retinal disease. Assessment of suitability for driving is usually by dynamic perimetry using a bowl perimeter.

Provocative tests for glaucoma

Some ophthalmologists put emphasis on provocative tests in doubtful cases of glaucoma. Angle closure may be 'provoked' by lying the patient prone in a darkened room for 45 min (prone darkroom test), or by dilating the pupils with certain combinations of mydriatic drugs (mydriatic test), noting the intraocular pressures before and after.

Patients with a tendency to glaucoma may show an increase of pressure after drinking a quantity of water (water drinking test).

Vascular imaging

Fluorescein angiography

The circulation within the eye and in the conjunctiva can be demonstrated by photography through suitable filters after the intravenous injection of sodium fluorescein. Fundus photography displays the retinal circulation and that of the underlying choroid.

This is a particularly sensitive way of demonstrating the changes in diabetic retinopathy (p. 91). It is also of value in assessing the extent of capillary closure in retinal vein thrombosis (p. 86) and thereby predicting the likelihood of secondary thrombotic glaucoma (p. 86). Prophylactic laser treatment is given if this risk is thought to be high.

Macular degenerations likely to benefit from laser treatment can be distinguished from the untreatable majority by fluorescein angiography (p. 90). This technique is also used to distinguish between true and pseudo-papilloedema, and between benign and malignant melanoma.

Intravenous fluorescein discolours the skin for a day or two and is excreted in the urine. It may cause transient nausea. In those with an allergic tendency more serious reactions, including laryngeal oedema and anaphylaxis, very rarely occur.

Carotid artery imaging

Doppler studies of the carotid blood flow are useful in the investigation of transient visual loss, without the hazards of angiography using contrast media.

Ultrasound

Ultrasonic waves, generated in a probe held in contact with the eye, are reflected by its structures, analysed and presented graphically on a screen. This is a non-invasive and painless technique.

A-scan

The probe is held in contact with the topically anaesthetized cornea and the echoes produced as the waves pass from one structure to another are measured. The most frequent use of the A-scan in ophthalmology is to determine the length of the eye prior to cataract surgery with the insertion of a lens implant. This measurement, combined with keratometry which gives a reading of the corneal curvature, allows an appropriate power of implant to be calculated and is termed 'biometry'.

B-scan

This allows the eye, optic nerve and orbit to be explored in any plane. Disorders of the posterior segment of the eye cap be detected even when cataract or other opacity, such as a vitreous haemorrhage, make visualization with an ophthalmoscope impossible. The technique is speedy and painless. A gel is used to establish contact between the probe and the closed eyelid.

Computerized tomography and nuclear magnetic resonance imaging

These imaging techniques are of value in demonstrating orbital and intracranial disease, complementing conventional radiology.

17. Visual standards

Screening of children for visual defects

The details of assessments of vision in apparently healthy children vary, but the following is a typical screening policy:

At 6 weeks screen for
- congenital cataract (red reflex)
- anatomical defects
- squint
- visual inattention (fixation and following).

At 18 months screen for squint (cover test).

At 3 years screen for
- squint (cover test)
- visual acuity (Stycar test at 3 m)
- refer if 3/6 or worse in either eye.

At school entry screen for
- squint (cover test)
- visual acuity (Sheridan Gardiner to Sonksen–Silver at 6 m)
- refer if 6/12 or less in either eye.

During school screen every other year with
- Snellen test type or other screening device (e.g. Keystone® screener)
- check for colour vision defect at 10 years.

Some children of school age who are disinclined to read, and whose educational achievements are unsatisfactory, are hypermetropic. The degree of hypermetropia may be insufficient to impair distance acuity, so the child passes a routine vision check, but reading is an effort. Children with reading difficulty should be referred for refraction.

Most teachers and parents are nowadays aware of the possibility that a child with reading or writing difficulties may be dyslexic. Specialist advice is available from educational psychologists.

Occupational visual standards

The visual standards set for employment in the services and in industry are complex. Advice may be obtained from the following United Kingdom sources, among others:

Army	Department of General Practice Royal Army Medical College Millbank, London (or local recruiting office)
British Airways	BA Medical Service Heathrow, London
British Rail	Regional Medical Officer at regional HQ
Dept of Transport	Driver and Vehicle Licensing Centre Swansea (includes HGV and PSV)
Merchant Navy	General Council of British Shipping Broomielaw Glasgow (or local Board of Trade examination centre)
RAF	Local recruiting office
Royal Navy	Department of General Practice Royal Naval Hospital Haslar, Gosport (or local recruiting office)

The principal visual criterion for employment is central visual acuity; colour vision is important in some jobs. There are variations between authorities as to whether the wearing of spectacles is permitted and, if so, of what strength.

In the UK, the following are the current requirements for drivers.

Department of Transport

Motor-car drivers

Vision tested on recognition of number plates. 'Slightly better than 6/12' is the nearest Snellen equivalent. Monocular vision no bar.

A driving licence may not be granted to a person suffering from some disability (including a disorder of the eye) which is likely to cause the driving of a vehicle by him to be a source of danger to the public.

Significant loss of visual field in both eyes — for example, homonymous hemianopia or advanced glaucoma — bars any form of driving licence, even if satisfactory central acuity is achieved.

The standards for visual acuity and visual fields are set by the Driver and Vehicle Licensing Centre at Swansea. In borderline cases a specialist opinion may be called for.

HGV and PSV

6/9 in the better, and 6/12 in the worse eye, corrected. Any pathological visual field defect is a bar. A 1981 standard for uncorrected static visual acuity of 6/60 in either eye separately is required.

18. Blindness and partial sight

The term 'blindness' does not necessarily imply total loss of sight. From the point of view of the social services, an individual is 'blind' when 'unable to perform any work for which eyesight is essential'. (Note — this definition does not mean 'unable to follow his previous occupation'.) In general, if the visual acuity is below 3/60 the above criterion is satisfied, though certain defects of the visual field may justify registration as 'blind' when the acuity is better than this.

Partial sightedness, although there is no statutory definition, is a condition in which substantial and permanent handicap exists, short of that requiring registration as 'blind'. This usually implies vision within the range 3/60 to 6/60, but coincident defects such as severe visual field loss may allow registration in the presence of visual acuity better than 6/60.

Registers of the blind and of the partially sighted are maintained by the social services departments in each area in the UK.

There follows a summary of the principal benefits available to those registered as handicapped on account of defective vision. The Social Work Department will provide assistance and advice, and it should be noted that some of the items listed are not available to the partially sighted, but only to the blind.

— Reduction in cost of TV licence
— Some travel concessions
— Postal concessions on articles for the blind
— Increased supplementary benefit, if applicable
— Blind person income tax relief
— Special visual aids, available through hospital eye service
— Advice on household management
— Education of visually handicapped children
— Training in Braille and other reading methods

— Hobbies and handicrafts
— Aids, appliances and games
— Talking books and tape recorders
— Large print books, from local libraries
— Training and rehabilitation in workshops for the blind.

Some useful addresses in the UK:

— Royal National Institute for the Blind
224 Great Portland Street
London WIN 6AA
— Partially Sighted Society
Queen's Road
Doncaster, S. Yorks DN1 2NX
(with branches in Exeter, London, and Wrexham;
among other functions, takes patients by direct referral for
free assessment of suitability for special visual aids).
— RNIB Talking Book Service for the Blind
Nuffield Library
Mount Pleasant
Wembley, Middlesex HA0 1RR
— British Wireless for the Blind Fund
34 New Road
Chatham ME4 4QR
(or contact through Social Services Dept)
— Telephone for the Blind Fund
Leigh
Nr Reigate
RH2 8RJ

The above-named bodies are among the many concerned with the education, training, employment and general welfare of those with visual handicap. There are many organizations and societies which have interests in particular areas or in sufferers from particular diseases. Among these are SENSE (The National Deaf, Blind, and Rubella Association), The British Diabetic Association, The Retinitis Pigmentosa Society, Guide Dogs for the Blind, and The Disabled Living Foundation.

The last-named body works to reduce the effects of disability by finding non-medical solutions to the daily living problems facing people of all ages with disabilities.

Details of the addresses, together with a summary of their respective aims and those of many other organizations, may be found in Charities Digest 1990, available in public libraries.

Glossary

Accommodation: The change in focus of the eye for clear viewing of near objects. Gradually diminishes with age with the development of presbyopia (q.v.).
Amblyopia: Visual defect in the absence of apparent disease (e.g. amblyopia of disuse, in squint).
Anterior chamber: Between cornea, in front, and iris and lens, behind.
Astigmatism: Irregular curvature of front surface of cornea, producing an aspherical surface. Can only be corrected by cylindrical lens or contact lens.
Blepharitis: Inflammation of the lid margins.
Cataract: Any opacity in the lens of the eye.
Chalazion: Meibomian cyst.
Chemosis: Oedema of the conjunctiva.
Choroid: The vascular coat of the eye, at the back.
Concomitant: Non-paralytic.
Cover test: The most important diagnostic test for squint.
Dacryocystitis: Inflammation of the tear sac.
Diplopia: Double vision.
Ectropion: Eversion of eyelid.
Emmetropia: The normal refractive state.
Entropion: Inversion of eyelid.
Epiphora: Watering of the eye.
Glaucoma: A collection of diseases characterised by elevation of the intraocular pressure.
Hemianopia: Loss of one half of the field of vision.
Heterophoria: Imbalance between the muscles of the two eyes, not amounting to actual squint.
Hordeolum: Stye.
Hypermetropia: Long-sight.
Hyphaema: Blood in the anterior chamber of the eye.

Keratoconus: Conical cornea.
'Lazy eye': Amblyopia following squint, etc
Limbus: Junction between cornea and sclera.
Miosis: Contraction of the pupil.
Mydriasis: Dilatation of the pupil.
Myopia: Short-sight.
Occlusion: Covering of an eye, usually to force the use of the other.
Ophthalmia neonatorum: Purulent conjunctivitis in infancy.
Orthophoria: Normal balance between the muscles of the two eyes.
Pinguecula: Conjunctival degenerative change at the limbus.
Proptosis: Exophthalmos.
Pterygium: A progressive opacity involving the cornea from the limbus.
Ptosis: Drooping of the upper lid.
Refraction: The state of focus of the eye. Also the estimation thereof.
Retinoblastoma: Malignant retinal tumour of childhood.
Retinopathy: Changes in the retina, usually reflecting systemic disease (e.g. hypertensive retinopathy).
Strabismus: Squint.
Sjögren's syndrome: A group of features associated with rheumatoid arthritis.
Sympathetic ophthalmia: Inflammatory changes affecting the second eye after a penetrating injury to the first.
Synechiae: Iris adhesions commonly following inflammation.
Trichiasis: Inturned eyelashes.
Uveitis: Inflammation of the iris, ciliary body, or choroid.
Xanthelasma: Creamy deposits in the skin; often of the lids.

Index

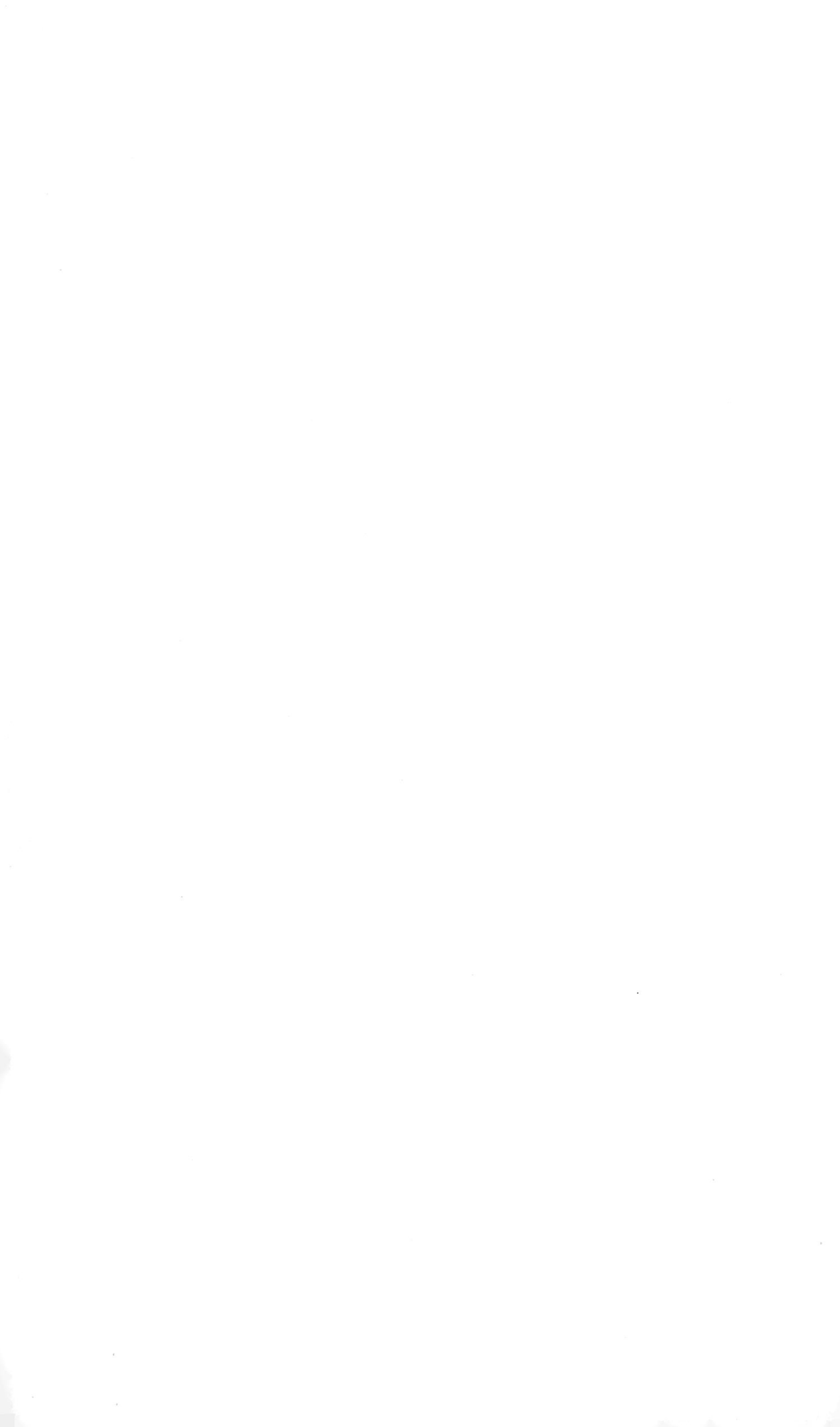